Fruitful

Fruitful

Cultivating a Spiritual Harvest That Won't Leave You Empty

Megan Hill and Melissa B. Kruger,
editors

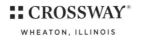

WHEATON, ILLINOIS

Fruitful: Cultivating a Spiritual Harvest That Won't Leave You Empty

© 2024 by Megan Hill and Melissa B. Kruger

Published by Crossway
   1300 Crescent Street
   Wheaton, Illinois 60187

Cover design: Crystal Courtney

First printing 2024

Printed in the United States of America

Trade paperback ISBN: 978-1-4335-9221-8
ePub ISBN: 978-1-4335-9223-2
PDF ISBN: 978-1-4335-9222-5

Library of Congress Cataloging-in-Publication Data

Names: Hill, Megan, 1978– editor. | Kruger, Melissa B., editor.

Title: Fruitful : cultivating a harvest that won't leave you empty / Megan Hill, Melissa B. Kruger, editors.

Description: Wheaton, Illinois : Crossway, [2024] | Series: Gospel coalition | Includes bibliographical references and index.

Identifiers: LCCN 2023029883 (print) | LCCN 2023029884 (ebook) | ISBN 9781433592218 (trade paperback) | ISBN 9781433592225 (pdf) | ISBN 9781433592232 (epub)

Subjects: LCSH: Christian women—Conduct of life. | Success—Religious aspects—Christianity. | Fruit of the Spirit. | Bible. Galatians, III, 22–23

Classification: LCC BV4527 .F78 2024 (print) | LCC BV4527 (ebook) | DDC 248.8/43—dc23/ eng/20231127

LC record available at https://lccn.loc.gov/2023029883

LC ebook record available at https://lccn.loc.gov/2023029884

Crossway is a publishing ministry of Good News Publishers.

VP   33 32 31 30 29 28 27 26 25 24
15 14 13 12 11 10 9 8 7 6 5 4 3 2 1

To the many women we've been able to meet
through the ministry of TGC.
We are so grateful for your kingdom service and the abundant
harvest the Lord is producing in and through you.

Contents

Introduction

How do you measure a successful life? Is it the number of likes or followers or double-taps? Is it the cleanliness of your kitchen or the letters after your name? Is it the sum of the things you've checked off your bucket list? Is it a sense of happiness or satisfaction? Is it what other people think about you?

Or is it something else entirely?

The Bible often uses the language of "fruitful" to describe a life well-lived. In the garden of Eden, God instructed our first parents to "be fruitful" (Gen. 1:28). In the Old Testament, he promised his people Israel that he would make them fruitful if they followed him (Lev. 26:9), and he pledged to restore them to fruitfulness when they disobeyed and repented (Jer. 23:3; Ezek. 36:11). Throughout the first books of the Bible, the good life is the fruitful life.

Even after the coming of Jesus, the Lord holds up fruitfulness as the measure of success for people who follow him. The New Testament is filled with encouragements to be fruitful. But instead of talking about fruitfulness in terms of abundant crops and large biological families, the Lord points his people to spiritual fruitfulness.

In the parable of the sower, Jesus describes the person whose heart is good soil, "who hears the word [of God] and understands it." This person "bears fruit and yields, in one case a hundredfold, in another sixty, and in another thirty" (Matt. 13:23). Although the metaphor is agricultural, Jesus's point is spiritual. A person who knows and receives the saving message of God's word will start to display the fruit of following Christ. If Christ is at work in your heart by his Spirit, your life will look different than it once did. Your life, in fact, will look a lot like Jesus.

Perhaps the most famous description of fruitfulness in the whole Bible comes from Galatians 5:22–25: "The fruit of the Spirit is love, joy, peace, patience, kindness, goodness, faithfulness, gentleness, self-control; against such things there is no law. And those who belong to Christ Jesus have crucified the flesh with its passions and desires. If we live by the Spirit, let us also keep in step with the Spirit."

In this devotional, we will look at each of the nine aspects of a fruitful life: love, joy, peace, patience, kindness, goodness, faithfulness, gentleness, and self-control. For each one, we will see how the Bible defines it, how Jesus displays it, what practicing it means for our own souls, and what it means for our relationships.

We'll be turning to a different passage of Scripture each day for forty days, since only the word of God can give us what we need for a fruitful life. As we do, we'll consider what that day's text has to say about bearing fruit in the power of the Spirit; we'll also look at additional Bible passages. It's not just one or two verses that can help us—it's the teaching of the whole Bible. Each section is capped off with one of our favorite fruit-filled recipes. We hope they will help you enjoy the sweetness of God's creation, reflect on his goodness, and share what you've learned with others.

You might choose to read this book on your own as part of your daily time of Bible reading and prayer, helping you to grow in your knowledge of God and love for him. But you might also want to read it with a friend or a group of friends, encouraging one another as you seek spiritual fruit in your lives together. Either way, the reflections, responses, and prayers that accompany each day's reading are designed to draw you closer to Christ as you display the fruit of walking with him.

Do you want a successful life? Come along with us as we ask for the Spirit's help to pursue a fruitful life.

Pursue a Better Dream

Melissa Kruger

Read

The fruit of the Spirit is love, joy, peace, patience, kindness, goodness, faithfulness, gentleness, self-control; against such things there is no law. And those who belong to Christ Jesus have crucified the flesh with its passions and desires. If we live by the Spirit, let us also keep in step with the Spirit. (Gal. 5:22–25)

Reflect

A few years ago, I read a book by a well-known influencer who encouraged her readers to build a "dream wall," a blank space to post images of their hopes for life, with specific goals they hoped to achieve. The dream wall would serve as a daily reminder of what each woman was working toward. If you could visualize it, the author promised, you could make it happen. The author's own dream wall included meeting famous people, being on the cover of influential magazines, and having a second home, in Hawaii.

The book left me with a sense of exhaustion and emptiness. It communicated: *Work harder, be better, do more, and you can achieve the life of your dreams!* The underbelly of that type of thinking is that if my life isn't living up to my dreams, it must be my fault. I also know enough about life (and my own heart) to recognize that I'd probably still be discontent even if I gained everything I think I want. A beach house in Hawaii isn't enough to satisfy a thirsty soul.

Today's verses point us to a different sort of dream wall. And, there's good news—the Spirit is the one doing the work. The Bible doesn't give us a message of work harder, do better. It gives us a message of dependence on Jesus: "I am the vine; you are the branches. Whoever abides in me and I in him, he it is that bears much fruit, for apart from me you can do nothing" (John 15:5). We flourish not by our own achievements, but by abiding in Jesus.

Instead of prioritizing earthly gains, the Spirit-filled dream wall imagines a fruit-bearing woman. The Spirit produces a singular fruit that blossoms in a beautiful variety of ways: love, joy, peace, patience, kindness, goodness, faithfulness, gentleness, and self-control. It's a different kind of hope from earthly gains. This spiritual dream wall offers a harvest that increases year to year. This fruit never spoils but offers a continual blessing to others. Whatever may happen outwardly, the inner soul is renewed and refreshed because the branches are abiding in the vine. This is an invitation to strive less and abide more.

It's also an encouragement to dream bigger. Take a moment to visualize an extravagant harvest of spiritual fruit. Ask God to make you joyful in every circumstance, patient with those who are difficult, gentle with those who make mistakes, and self-controlled when life feels out of control. This is the fruit of a soul that abides in Jesus. As we walk by his Spirit, he teaches us more about himself and then produces fruit that reflects Jesus in our lives.

Respond

In what ways do earthly gains and successes tend to leave us always wanting more? What would it look like for you to prioritize abiding in Jesus in the hopes of bearing spiritual fruit?

Request

O Lord, I want to be like Jesus. Fill me with your Spirit and transform me by your word. As I abide in you, bear your fruit through me. Let me be filled with love, joy, peace, patience, kindness, goodness, faithfulness, gentleness, and self-control. Let me be blessed to be a blessing as I keep in step with the Spirit.

LOVE

Let me tell you where love was born. Love was born in the garden of Gethsemane, where Jesus sweat great drops of blood, it was nurtured in Pilate's hall, where Jesus bared his back to the ploughing of the lash, and gave his body to be spit upon and scourged. Love was nurtured at the cross, amid the groans of an expiring God, beneath the droppings of his blood—it was there that love was nurtured. Bear me witness, children of God. Where did your love spring from, but from the foot of the cross?

CHARLES SPURGEON[1]

Love Begins with God

Abbey Wedgeworth

Read

The Lord passed before him and proclaimed, "The Lord, the Lord, a God merciful and gracious, slow to anger, and abounding in steadfast love and faithfulness, keeping steadfast love for thousands, forgiving iniquity and transgression and sin." (Ex. 34:6–7)

Reflect

What is love?

I can't ask that question without the 1990s Haddaway song popping into my mind. And now I'm sitting here in a coffee shop, bobbing my head to the beat: "What is love? Baby, don't hurt me." But the lyrics that follow this iconic intro do nothing to answer that question. Perhaps a better song title would be "What Isn't Love?"

The Bible offers more concrete definitions. In 1 Corinthians 13 (the frontrunner for the superlative "Most likely to be read at a wedding"), the apostle Paul explicitly answers the question, What is love? It is patient and kind. It isn't self-seeking. It bears and believes all things. It doesn't envy, and it doesn't end. In his New Testament letter, John provides an even more poignant and concise definition: "God is love" (1 John 4:8, 16). Before time, love existed between Father, Son, and Spirit. Man was made in God's image as an overflow of that Trinitarian love. His definition reveals the history of love and also its source: God.

Because we are his image bearers, we have the ability to love as he loves.

The English word for *love* is a little sloppy. I *love* my nail polish. I also *love* my child. The word communicates affection in both contexts but only self-sacrificial care in the latter. We can usually discern the difference based on the context. However, in the Bible, numerous Greek and Hebrew words for love offer us categories for different types of love, leaving less room for misunderstanding.

There is sexual love (*eros/yada*), friendship love (*phileo/ahabah*), and familial love (*storge/ahabah*). But the most common word for love used in the Greek portion of the Bible is *agape*. It refers to charity, love that is unchanged regardless of changing circumstances. *Agape's* Hebrew counterpart is *hesed*, which refers to steadfast love or lovingkindness. This word is most commonly used to describe God's love for his people in the Old Testament.

In the first description of his attributes found in the Bible, God says he abounds in steadfast love (Ex. 34:6–7). Shockingly, God isn't saying this to nice people who follow him faithfully. He says it to destructive and self-seeking people. To them, he describes himself as overflowing with forgiveness, kindness, and commitment.

Just as Paul defines love by what it does and does not do, and John exhorts Christians to love, not just in word but also in deed (1 John 3:18), God's description of himself shows that love is never merely affection—it is *action*. The ultimate demonstration of love in action is God's love for us in Christ Jesus. In love, God preserves his people. In love, he gives us his Son. In love, he pours out his Spirit. And his Spirit enables us to respond according to the commands he has given us—in *love*.

This sort of love is not natural. Without the Spirit, we love people the way I love my nail polish. Love becomes a matter of preference or performance. But what happens when our preferences change? What about when people no longer meet our needs or please us? By contrast, God's love—steadfast love—endures all things. His love is different from our love.

As beloved of God, those who love him receive the ability to love as he does through the power of his Spirit. To define love, we need to know its source. To practice love, we need the God who *is* love to live in us.

Respond

If you were asked by a stranger on the street how you define love, how would you respond? What experiences have most shaped your understanding of love? How do your experiences compare or contrast with the definitions offered in 1 Corinthians 13:1–13 and 1 John 3:16–20?

Request

Father, I praise you that you are a God who is merciful and gracious, slow to anger, and abounding in steadfast love and

faithfulness. I am in awe of how you forgive iniquity and transgression and sin. I am humbled to be a recipient of your mercy,
grace, patience, forgiveness, and steadfast love. Thank you for your
faithfulness to me, even when I am faithless. Forgive me for the
times I fail to show love. Please convict me when I am not loving
well, and help me by the power of your Spirit to love others as
you have loved me.

Love Came Down

Abbey Wedgeworth

Read

As the Father has loved me, so have I loved you. Abide in my
love. . . . This is my commandment, that you love one another
as I have loved you. Greater love has no one than this, that
someone lay down his life for his friends. (John 15:9–13)

Reflect

Algebra wasn't my favorite subject, but it's served me well in
learning about love. Do you remember the transitive property?
It's the one that says, if A = B and B = C, then A = C. So, if A = 5,
for example, then B and C must both also be 5 by the transitive
property.

God is love. And Christ is God. Therefore, Christ is love. So
if you want to know what love is, and what love does, look no
further than the life of Christ. He provided a living, breathing,
walking, talking definition of love.

He spent his life welcoming the shunned, touching the untouchable, enduring the folly and failure of his friends, healing the sick, and defending the vulnerable. All of these led to his pinnacle display of love: he laid down his life for us.

That's why his invitation to "love one another as I have loved you" in John 15 is such a tall order. How has he loved us? To the point of death.

We cannot heed the command to love without receiving the invitation to abide. Jesus's call for us to abide—to remain—in his love is really an equipping to fulfill his otherwise impossible command. In the greatest display of love there has ever been and ever will be, he gave his life for us. And now, he invites us to join him in the work of loving others.

Love may not require us to be nailed to a cross or jump in front of a moving vehicle to save someone else, but it almost always involves death of some sort. It might look like dying to pride or retribution by saying, "I forgive you, and I will not hold it against you." Or perhaps it looks like dying to ambition or appetite to let another go first. Maybe it looks like dying to the desire to have the last word for the sake of peace. Perhaps it looks like risking your own health to care for someone who is sick and ailing.

We cannot love sacrificially on our own. Paul Miller writes, "You simply do not have the power or wisdom or ability in yourself to love. You know without a shadow of a doubt that you can't love. That is the beginning of faith—knowing you can't love. Faith is the power for love."[2] Jesus must be more than our example of how to love, he must empower our love.

My campus pastor used to say that Christianity is a race to the bottom. Jesus condescended to us by leaving glory to take on flesh. He stooped low over and over in his earthly life out of love for others, washing feet and serving those who would fail and betray him. But Jesus never asks us to go lower than he was willing to go himself. He's our running mate all the way down, and he's the prize at the end of that gloriously worthwhile race that ends in resurrection life.

Hollywood would lead us to believe that love is the most natural, carefree feeling in the world. But the Bible reveals that true love often feels more like self-denial than self-actualization. It often feels like death. But Jesus also showed us that Christian love is the sort of death that leads to resurrection life. The same power that raised him from the dead, his Spirit, lives in us, empowering us through his grace to love as he loved, straight to the bottom, all the way to glory.

Respond

How is Christ's example of love a source of encouragement to you today? In what circumstances do you sometimes resist the call to love sacrificially like your Savior?

Request

Jesus, by your life you provided a model for love. In your death you atoned for my failure to love. In your resurrection you made it possible for me to love. Would you empower me by your Spirit to love like you do? Help me to clearly discern the places you are calling me to die to myself out of love for others. In those moments, bring to mind your steadfast love and cause me to feel near to you in that place. Then would you, by your grace, give me eyes to see the fruit of resurrection life in my heart and relationships? Do it for your glory, I ask.

Love Changes Everything

Abbey Wedgeworth

Read

In this is love, not that we have loved God but that he loved us
and sent his Son to be the propitiation for our sins. Beloved,
if God so loved us, we also ought to love one another. No one
has ever seen God; if we love one another, God abides in us
and his love is perfected in us. (1 John 4:10–12)

Reflect

I remember the first time my (now) husband, David, told me he
loved me. We sat in his black Ford F-150 overlooking a mountain
range. When my gaze met his, which turned my head from the
view like a magnet, he just blurted it out: "I love you." He had
driven me up here to tell me. I looked into those sincere blue eyes
I had seen for the first time only four weeks earlier and replied
matter-of-factly, "No, you don't." And I proceeded to list every
terrible thing I could think of about myself.

People often say about love, "When you know, you know." But David said to me, "When you decide, you decide. And I've decided. You're my choice, and I won't leave you."

In Romans 5:6–8, Paul describes the revelation of God's love for us in that while we were still sinners, while we were still weak, Christ died for us, the ungodly. There is no merit on our part. Though we brought nothing good to the table, God set his love on us. He set his self-sacrificial, unconditional, steadfast love on us. "This is love: not that we loved God, but that he loved us and sent his Son to be the propitiation for our sins" (1 John 4:10).

Being loved like this changes everything. His love offers us cleansing, acceptance, and security. He pulls us out of a chaotic quest for our needs to be met, and in meeting them, fills us to overflowing to meet the needs of others. That overflow means that this identity shift is also a vocational shift. "We love because he first loved us," explains 1 John 4:19. Rather than walking into every encounter with others as if we are applying for a job, we walk in to *do* a job. As one who is loved by God, we love. John makes it clear in today's passage that if we love God, we will love others, and furthermore, that if we do not love, we don't know God.

John, who refers to himself as the one whom Jesus loved, also here highlights three benefits of practicing love. First, it offers assurance of salvation (vv. 7–8). Loving others demonstrates God's work in our lives. Second, although we can't see God, love offers us evidence of his presence with us. Loving is about as close to seeing God as we can get this side of glory (v. 12). Lastly, as we practice love, God's love is perfected within us (v. 12). Loving others makes us more like our loving God.

The beauty of being secure in the love of God is that we are free from riding the roller coaster of the approval of others. As we look to the interests of others (rather than our own), we are free from the plague of disappointment. As we forgive others, we are free from the tyranny of bitterness. But more than that, we carry refreshment everywhere we go. As we seek to love others— by imitating God and empowered by his love—we invite others to taste and see that the Lord is good.

Respond

In what ways do you live as someone who is trying to earn God's love? How do the verses from today encourage you specifically? Can you think of a time when your identity as "loved by God" fueled your love for someone who felt impossible to love?

Request

Father, I have spiritual amnesia. I so quickly forget the reality that I am loved by you. I fall back into the habits of seeking approval from others and even trying to prove myself to you. Please increase my faith in the reality of your love for me. Let me be a refreshment to others for your glory and for their good. Thank you for setting your love on me.

Let Love Be Genuine

Abbey Wedgeworth

Read

Let love be genuine. Abhor what is evil; hold fast to what is good. Love one another with brotherly affection. Outdo one another in showing honor. (Rom. 12:9–10)

Reflect

About a decade ago, I traveled with two friends to help one of them clean out her mom's things after her mother's death. We hadn't been friends long, and this scenario was an honor. Over and over throughout the trip, however, I found myself often literally, and sometimes figuratively, in the back seat, while the other friend sat in a more privileged position.

Sadly, the verses from today always remind me of this trip. I wanted credit for what I was doing, and I was resentful of not getting to play the role that I wanted to in my friend's grief. I was willing to offer myself and my services, but my motivation was selfish. I wanted closer friendship. I wanted intimacy. Because my goal was not love, and I was filled with concern for myself instead of for her, I got the opposite of what I intended: loneliness and bitterness.

In Romans 12, Paul tells the church how believers are to treat one another, urging them, "Let love be genuine." He sets the tone for this passage by reminding them of their position in Christ: "by the mercies of God" Paul says that God's love for us in Christ is the foundation for how we are to treat one another. In Jesus, we are fully accepted, fully loved, and fully equipped. The gospel causes us to stop viewing people as pawns to manipulate to serve our own needs and to start seeing them as image bearers whom we can love and serve. True love is too fixated on Jesus to be filled with thoughts of self.

This call to genuine love has profound implications for our families, our churches, and the watching world. Love forges diverse friendships, preserves marriages in the face of disappointment, protects children, restores people to the truth, reconciles relationships after misunderstanding or wrongdoing, welcomes the marginalized and outcast, and demonstrates a countercultural way of living that ensures people will know that we are Christians by our love. And the love we have for the lost leads us to practice radical hospitality, welcoming those who are different from us.

Our position in Christ changes our posture toward one another. Rather than looking at others with thoughts of self—*How can you help me? How can you make me look good? How can you make me feel good? How can I use you to feel more secure?*—we ask God, *How do you want me to share your love with this person? How can*

I encourage and support her? What does she need from me? We move toward others with a self-forgetful love.

The way our hearts respond to others reveals our understanding of God's love for us in Christ Jesus. But if you're falling short, be encouraged. As I recognized my failure to love my grieving friend well and in turn felt insecure and unlovable, God's love for me felt even more amazing and undeserved. He exposed my unbelief and his sufficiency. When you fail to love well, you too have the chance to see more clearly the nature of God's steadfast love for you.

Believe in him. Be loved by him. And watch the fruit grow.

Respond

Think of a person with whom you are either regularly disappointed or often annoyed. How might your next interaction look different if you responded to her out of genuine love?

Request

Father, I confess that I am often impatient and unkind. I am filled with envy and often boast. I am arrogant and claim the moral high ground. I am rude when inconvenienced. I often insist on my own way, considering myself more important than others. I grow irritable and resentful, keeping a record of wrongs so that I can be right, which often keeps me from being connected. Sometimes my love is lazy and sentimental instead of truth-filled and honest. I know that if I do not have love, I am nothing. Help me, by your Spirit, Lord, to believe in your love and to love others well.

Best-Ever Raspberry Muffins

Courtney Doctor

I used to make these with my (future) mother-in-law when I was dating my (future) husband.

Makes 12 muffins or 1 loaf
Preheat oven to 400 degrees

Ingredients

- 1½ cups all-purpose flour
- ½ teaspoon baking soda
- ½ teaspoon salt
- 1½ teaspoons ground cinnamon
- 1 cup sugar
- 1 12-ounce package frozen unsweetened raspberries, thawed
- 2–3 eggs, well beaten
- ½ cup vegetable oil
- ½ cup chopped pecans (optional, but really good!)

Instructions

- Mix flour, baking soda, salt, cinnamon, and sugar.

- Make a well in the center and stir in undrained raspberries and eggs. Stir in oil and pecans.

- Spoon batter into lightly greased muffin tins (muffin cups will be full, but the batter is heavy and will not overflow).

- Bake 15–20 minutes. Cool 5 minutes before removing from pan.

- Note: The batter can also be baked in a greased and floured 9 x 5–inch loaf pan at 350 degrees for 1 hour or until a wooden pick inserted in center comes out clean.

JOY

Let us, then, seek not the stream, but the fountain;
not primarily the joy, but that real and living
union with Jesus by which His joy becomes ours.

FRANCES RIDLEY HAVERGAL[3]

True Joy Doesn't Fade

Lydia Brownback

Read

You make known to me the path of life;
   in your presence there is fullness of joy;
   at your right hand are pleasures forevermore. (Ps. 16:11)

Reflect

Birthday parties, bridal showers, holiday feasts—despite the stress about details, decisions, and inevitable glitches, we plan and prepare for these occasions with delight-fueled energy. Party day finally comes, and it's such fun to watch the fruit of our labors give pleasure to others.

Afterward, when the guests have left and the cleanup is done, we expect to put our feet up and bask in a sense of well-being, but sometimes, much to our surprise, we feel a bit blue instead, as the thought creeps in—*Now what?* All those weeks of happy anticipation—over and done in a few short hours. These day-after blues remind us that nothing in this life—even the best things—brings unfading joy. That kind of joy—the deep, abiding joy that the psalmist expresses in Psalm 16—has a completely different source.

The author of Psalm 16, King David, was no stranger to life's ups and downs. He had a lot of royal privileges and material blessings, but none of that kept him from troubles, trials, and threats to his very own life. In the midst of it all, he came to know the Lord his God. And because he experienced the Lord's faithfulness in both good times and bad, he'd learned not to base his well-being on his circumstances. His life lessons led him to declare with heartfelt conviction, "The LORD is my chosen portion" (v. 5). David knew he was safe in God's care, so he anchored his life in God's words and ways, "the path of life" God had shown him (v. 11). That's why his well-being didn't rise and fall with the peaks and valleys. Through the various ups and downs, he could say, "The lines have fallen for me in pleasant places; indeed, I have a beautiful inheritance" (v. 6).

The words of this psalm reflect true joy, the fruit of a God-centered life. "I have set the LORD always before me," David declares, "because he is at my right hand, I shall not be shaken" (v. 8). Deep, abiding, unfading joy is never found in our circumstances—not even in the happiest of special occasions or successes or milestones. It's found only in God's presence and in the path of life marked out for us by God in his word.

Psalm 16 shows us that a God-centered life brings joy because it's only by centering on God that we can truly know him as he is—kind, loving, merciful, gracious, and mighty to save. David knew from personal experience that the Lord was his refuge (v. 1), and that's why joy defined him. But this deep, steady joy isn't reserved for God-appointed kings like David or for those Christians who seem to have their spiritual act together. Real joy is Spirit-grown fruit that ripens in our hearts as we abide in our Savior, shape our day-to-day lives by his word, commune with him in prayer, and surround ourselves with sisters and brothers in Christ.

What we need more than podcasts and seminars that offer us ten tips to a better spiritual life (helpful as they might be) is simply to make the Lord the center of everything, to anchor our priorities, plans, and purposes in his ways and words. As we do, we are characterized more and more by joy—true joy that doesn't fade when the party is over.

Respond

Jot down the specific attitudes, outlooks, and actions David expresses in Psalm 16. How do you think each of these brings about personal well-being and steady joy in all the ups and downs of life? Which one speaks most deeply to your heart, and why?

Request

Lord, I confess that too often I chase worldly happiness instead of the fullness of joy that comes from belonging to Christ. Please open my eyes to see that what you hold out to me in Christ is so much richer than anything this world offers. I want to know you as my portion, my refuge. Enlarge my view of you so that fullness of joy can be mine at all times. I welcome your transforming work, Lord, because by it you enlarge my capacity to see you as you are and to rejoice in the truth that I am yours and you are mine forever.

Jesus Has This

Lydia Brownback

Read

> Therefore, since we are surrounded by so great a cloud of witnesses, let us also lay aside every weight, and sin which clings so closely, and let us run with endurance the race that is set before us, looking to Jesus, the founder and perfecter of our faith, who for the joy that was set before him endured the cross, despising the shame, and is seated at the right hand of the throne of God. (Heb. 12:1–2)

Reflect

"You got this!" When we need a shot of encouragement, this empowerment slogan is readily available on everything from greeting cards to GIFs. The problem is, it's just not true. We simply can't manage life's struggles in our own strength, whether it's sickness or broken relationships or entrenched patterns of sin. We try and fail. So we dust ourselves off and go at it with fresh zeal, only to be confronted again, sooner or later, with the reality of our inadequacy. At this point, we have a choice. We can give in to discouragement, or we can lift our eyes off our problems and onto Jesus.

Jesus faced the greatest struggle anyone has ever faced—suffering on the cross to bear God's righteous wrath against sin. Before him lay the unspeakable anguish of God's judgment, which he would experience on behalf of sinners like you and me. So he fell on his knees and prayed, "Father, if you are willing, remove this cup from me." So great was his angst about the approaching ordeal that "his sweat became like great drops of blood falling down to the ground." But afterward he got up to face the suffering, having also prayed, "Nevertheless, not my will, but yours, be done" (Luke 22:42–44). What enabled him to endure? It was joy. He endured the cross "for the joy that was set before him" (Heb. 12:2). Jesus looked beyond the immediate, short-term pain to the never-ending joy on the other side of it, and this focus strengthened him to endure.

We can endure our own hardships and challenges—not because we've "got this" but because Jesus did. The author of Hebrews tells us in today's verses that endurance comes not by gritting our teeth and trying harder but by looking at Jesus. As we look at him, we find that we actually can lay aside the "weight" of discouragement and the sins that pull us down again and again. And much to our surprise, we find our joy increasing. Joy is inevitable as we focus on the actual source of joy. It's what equips us to more easily reject our pet sins and unhelpful coping devices. We realize we don't need them anymore, and we never actually did.

Sooner or later, our pain will end, but the joy held out to us in Jesus never will. He's got this!

Respond

What weights and sins are keeping you stuck and joyless? Hebrews shows us that the ability to make seemingly impossible changes begins by looking at Jesus. We find him on every page of God's word. We meet him in prayer. We meet him in worship and in the particular body of believers where he's placed us. This is how we look at Jesus. What practical changes can you make in your life to enlarge your view of him?

Request

Thank you, Jesus, for enduring the cross to pay for my sins and bind me to you forever. I get so easily drawn away from you by my difficulties, not to mention the little daily cares and pressures, and then I find myself turning to worldly comforts to cope. Please help me to lift my gaze off myself and my life and all its clutter to see you as my joyful Savior. As I do, please increase my capacity for joy so I'll reflect you more and more as I live each day.

Find Joy When Life Hurts

Lydia Brownback

Read

> Though the fig tree should not blossom,
>   nor fruit be on the vines,
> the produce of the olive fail
>   and the fields yield no food,
> the flock be cut off from the fold
>   and there be no herd in the stalls,
> yet I will rejoice in the LORD;
>   I will take joy in the God of my salvation.
> GOD, the Lord, is my strength;
>   he makes my feet like the deer's;
>   he makes me tread on my high places. (Hab. 3:17–19)

Reflect

A fictional orphan girl named Pollyanna still captivates young readers, even though her story was written more than a century ago. Pollyanna lived with a stern spinster aunt who treated her harshly, but the young orphan survived by looking for something good in every bad situation. A cheerful outlook like Pollyanna's does lift our spirits, but it's not the same as joy—the deep, settled, Spirit-given joy that has nothing to do with finding bits and pieces of positivity during hard days. The joy the Spirit gives isn't found through teeth-gritting determination and a pasted-on smile.

Habakkuk the prophet saw nothing sunny and bright on the horizon. In fact, the Lord revealed to him that great trouble and loss lay ahead. The Lord was going to come and severely discipline his people for their unrepentant sin. The prophet made no attempt to put a positive spin on this frightening news. Instead, he was honest about his fear (v. 16). But it's right there, where he could see nothing but present gloom and future doom, that Habakkuk chose to rejoice. Despite how the Lord's plan was making him feel, the prophet determined to dwell on all he knew about the character of God.

It's easy to rejoice in the Lord when we have every expectation of a happy outcome or when a long-awaited answer to prayer finally comes. But rejoicing when there seems to be no answer, or when we don't like the answer we receive, can be a lot harder. What enabled Habakkuk to rejoice when bad news came? For one thing, he knew God's good promises to his people. When violence and destruction surrounded him, he reflected on the truth about God, which renewed his joy and strengthened his faith. Habakkuk's fear was very real, but he didn't turn away from the Lord. Instead he chose to accept what the Lord revealed to him. From this prophet, we glimpse the power of joy.

When we really trust God, no matter how bad things seem, we can do what Habakkuk did—bow before God's will and choose joy. If we do, we too will find the strength that joy gives us to tread on high places.

Respond

How do you respond when bad news comes or when your circumstances don't match your expectations? If we want to be joy-filled women, we must be willing to accept God's ways in our lives, even when they don't seem to make sense. And sometimes we choose to rejoice even when we don't feel joyful. In what situation or area of your life can you apply Habakkuk's response of faith, and how might this change you, even if your circumstances remain the same?

Request

Heavenly Father, humble my heart to accept your plan for me and to respond with joyful praise. I pray for eyes to see you as you truly are—faithful, kind, powerful, and worthy of my unreserved trust in your goodness. I want to know the strength that accompanies rejoicing so that I'll know the love of my Savior and live through him for your glory and my joy.

Rejoice Always

Lydia Brownback

Read

Rejoice in the Lord always; again I will say, rejoice. Let your reasonableness be known to everyone. The Lord is at hand; do not be anxious about anything, but in everything by prayer and supplication with thanksgiving let your requests be made known to God. And the peace of God, which surpasses all understanding, will guard your hearts and your minds in Christ Jesus. (Phil. 4:4–7)

Reflect

"Rejoice," the apostle Paul instructs, and keep on rejoicing. We find this encouragement all through his letter to the Philippians, even though he penned his words from a prison cell. How we respond to difficulty speaks volumes to a watching world about the Lord we profess to follow. Rejoicing in seasons of disappointment or hardship communicates that what we have *in* the Lord is so much better than the earthly blessings we get *from* the Lord. And it communicates that he is trustworthy.

The immediate context of Paul's call to rejoice was a disagreement between Euodia and Syntyche, two women in the church at Philippi who weren't getting along. We aren't told why these women fell out, but our inability to know the specifics enables us to apply Paul's words to our own relational conflicts, whatever they might be. The particulars always differ, but whatever the cause of the conflict, we want to guard ourselves against a competitive spirit, the kind that kicks in when the position, pleasure, or power we crave feels threatened. Competitiveness can creep into our relationships at home, at work, or at church, and it can show up in our cyber life, as we vie for clicks and likes and follows on social media platforms. We want a seat at the table—and sometimes not just any seat, but a prominent one. We want to count, to have our opinion or our contribution matter. But the truth is, there's no real joy in getting that place at the table or being proven right or coming out on top. Winning isn't what makes life worth living.

Because our present and our future are secure in Christ, we can be reasonable. In him, we've already been given everything we will ever need. So we don't have to be proven right. We don't have to strive for top position—or any position. We don't have to fight for blessing. The Lord is at hand in your life and mine, and we can be sure that the plans, purposes, and provision appointed for us will surely come. That's why rejoicing is always reasonable. It's why we can love and serve our brothers and sisters in Christ rather than compete with them. It's why joy can define our life and relationships.

And whenever conflict threatens to arise and sabotage our joy, we can pray. As Paul notes, we have an open invitation to tell God all our longings, fears, hopes, and concerns. The answers we receive might differ from what we hoped or thought we needed, but we can be sure they're even better. "If God is for us, who can be against us? He who did not spare his own Son but gave him up for us all, how will he not also with him graciously give us all things?" (Rom. 8:31–32). Because this is true, we can rejoice and rejoice and rejoice some more. In light of all we have in Christ—both now and forever—joy is always reasonable.

Respond

Paul's command to "rejoice in the Lord always" was written from prison. How has your faith been encouraged by someone who chose to rejoice in spite of a difficult situation? How could you choose to rejoice in the Lord in the midst of the various trials in your life today?

Request

My precious Lord, I am reminded today that you, the Creator God of the world and everything in it, take note of the details of my life and are always at work in them. Because that's true, I have no reason to be anxious and every reason to rejoice. I pray to live with conscious awareness of your loving care so that joy will define me and shape the way I relate to the people you've given me to love.

Mama Too's Summer Peach Pie

Courtney Doctor

This was my grandmother's (Mama Too's) recipe. My niece and I make it every summer in her honor.

Preheat oven to 350 degrees

Ingredients

- 1 unbaked pie crust
- ¾ cup sugar
- 4 tablespoons flour
- 3 tablespoons cinnamon
- ½ pint heavy whipping cream
- Sliced fresh (ripe) peaches, enough to fill the pie shell

Instructions

- Mix sugar, flour, and cinnamon together in a small bowl.

- Spread half of mixture on the bottom of pie crust. Put enough sliced peaches in to fill the crust.

- Pour cream over the top and sprinkle the rest of the sugar mixture over all. Bake at 350 for 45 minutes.

- Cool for 20 minutes before putting in fridge. Let refrigerate for 24 hours.

PEACE

True peace comes not from the absence of
trouble but from the presence of God.

ALEXANDER MACLAREN[4]

God Designed You for Peace

Courtney Doctor

Read

The LORD bless you and keep you;
the LORD make his face to shine upon you and be gracious
to you;
the LORD lift up his countenance upon you and give you
peace. (Num. 6:24–26)

Reflect

What brings you peace? A quick scroll through social media reveals multiple attempts at answering that question. Some indicate that peace is a commodity we gain while sitting by a quiet lake, strolling on a wooded path, or gazing at the night sky. Others imply that a sparkling clean kitchen, a freshly made bed, a basket of folded laundry, or an inbox clear of unanswered emails will garner peace in your life. And most of us have probably said (or at least thought), "All I want is a little peace and quiet." What we mean is, we want a quiet afternoon. And to be honest, who wouldn't love a quiet day? Most of us would be happy with a few quiet moments! But is peace merely the absence of noise, the result of completed tasks, or something only to be found when our environment is beautiful?

No. The Bible presents the idea of peace as something much greater, much more holistic, and much more beneficial than merely a quiet afternoon. The Hebrew word for peace is *shalom*. And *shalom* is something that is meant to permeate every aspect of a person's life with wholeness, goodness, and well-being. It's the true peace we all long for because it's the peace God designed us for.

We see this perfect peace in the first two chapters of the Bible— in Eden. During this time and in this place, Adam and Eve were able to walk with God in unbroken fellowship. They experienced what it was to be in God's presence and, as a result, knew true peace with God, each other, and all of creation. They experienced *shalom* and, consequently, true human flourishing.

But because of Adam and Eve's rebellion, they became enemies of God and were cast out of Eden, losing both their access to this place of perfect *shalom* and their perfect union with the God of *shalom*. However, today's verses show us that God still longs to give his people peace.

Did you notice how many times the Lord is mentioned? Three times; at the beginning of each part of the blessing. The gifts that God gives—protection, provision, and peace—will never be given apart from him. God longs to give, not just the gifts we seek, but himself. It's only in his presence that we will find peace.

In today's verses, we're told that God "makes his face shine on" us and "lifts his countenance upon" us. Both mean that God looks on us with joy, love, and delight. The expression on his face is that of a loving parent gazing on the child he adores. As scholar Jay Sklar wrote, "This intimate language describes the Lord turning his face to us, beaming with love and pleasure. That is true blessing: the King of the universe looking towards you as a loving Father who knows all your needs and giving you his very self."[5] What deeper source of peace could we ever find than the holy, infinite, majestic, Creator God looking on us with love and joy?

True peace is available. It's available because we serve a loving God. Peace is available because, ultimately, God sent his Son, the Prince of Peace, to accomplish all that's required to give us peace. As you consider the ways you search for peace in your life, remember that true peace is greater, deeper, and better than merely a quiet moment or two. Peace is the gift of God given to his children when they are brought back into right relationship with him and can, once again, live in his presence.

Respond

Where do you turn to find peace? What kind of peace do you long for? What is the relationship between God's countenance and peace?

Request

Father, thank you that you are a God of peace. Thank you that you reconcile your children to yourself and give us your peace. Help me look to you as the only source of true and lasting peace.

You Need Two Kinds of Peace

Courtney Doctor

Read

Peace I leave with you; my peace I give to you. Not as the world gives do I give to you. Let not your hearts be troubled, neither let them be afraid. (John 14:27)

Reflect

I once saw a bumper sticker that read, "No Jesus—No Peace; Know Jesus—Know Peace." I'm not a big fan of bumper-sticker theology, but this one was right. Apart from Jesus, it is impossible to know real peace—deep, genuine, lasting peace. But because of Jesus, the Prince of Peace, we can!

There are two types of peace we all need: peace *with* God and the peace *of* God. Peace with God is the peace made between God and his enemies. Because of the rebellion against God in the garden, all humans are born in a state of conflict with God, and there's nothing we can do to end the war. In fact, we continue to make war against God. But God so loved the world that he sent his only Son to reconcile us to God (John 3:16). When we trust in Christ and are united to him, he grants us peace with God.

After we have peace *with* God, Jesus freely gives us the peace *of* God. This is the gift of peace that our hearts long for, the one that enables us to live peacefully in the moments of our days. When Jesus spoke the words of today's verse to his disciples, it was the night before the crucifixion, and Jesus had just told them he was going away. They were confused, frightened, and feeling abandoned. So Jesus gave them the gift of peace.

Paul wrote in Philippians 4:7 that "the peace of God, which surpasses all understanding, will guard your hearts and your minds in Christ Jesus." Jesus offered his disciples the power of peace, then and now. It transcends all understanding—meaning, it doesn't always make sense. It defies our circumstances. It guards our hearts amid sorrow and suffering and our minds during chaos and confusion. It can protect our emotions from spinning out of control and our thoughts from racing. The peace of Jesus steadies us when our circumstances shake us.

Peace is the fruit of prayer, given through the Holy Spirit. We don't find this peace through self-help books or by thinking positive thoughts. We don't get this peace through enlightenment or empty meditation. We receive this peace from the only one who can give it. The Lord gives strength to his people and blesses them with peace (Ps. 29:11). In the midst of all of our trials and tribulations, this is an amazing blessing from the Lord.

Respond

Describe a time when you either experienced the peace that passes all understanding (Phil. 4:7) or saw it in someone else's life. Why do you think we can only experience the peace *of* God after we've been granted peace *with* God?

Request

Father, thank you that you have made a way for us to be at peace with you. And thank you that you bless us with your peace. Please grant me this peace that passes all understanding, and may it guard my heart and mind at all times.

Peace Comes from Trust

Courtney Doctor

Read

You keep him in perfect peace
  whose mind is stayed on you,
  because he trusts in you. (Isa. 26:3)

Reflect

I used to own the most anxious horse that ever walked this planet. She was fidgety and scared of almost everything. When she encountered new sights or new obstacles, she would huff at them and try to flee. Whether I was riding her or walking next to her, I would attempt to reassure her and give her time to adjust. But at the end of the day, I just wanted her to trust me and move over, through, or around the obstacle in her way.

How many of us go through life the same way? We live in constant fear and anxiety. New situations come at us, and we want to flee. When I owned this horse, I repeatedly saw how much I was like her and how God wanted no less from me than I wanted from her—to trust him and move forward in peace. It's what he wants for all of us.

In today's verse, Isaiah makes a connection between peace and trust. Peace is for those who trust God, and those who trust God will have peace. And it's not hard to see why. We all trust in something. If we want to have peace in life's sufferings and sorrows, then whatever we trust in must be stronger than the trial we face. Only God is stronger than anything in this life. Only God is wise enough to see you through. Only God is able to hold you no matter what threatens to undo you. Only God can keep you in perfect peace.

But how does it happen? How do we receive that kind of peace and cultivate that kind of trust? It's captured in the phrase "whose mind is stayed on you." The battle for peace is waged in our mind. Paul told the Corinthian believers that we are engaged in a spiritual battle, and we fight this battle by taking "every thought captive to obey Christ" (2 Cor. 10:5). One of the most important spiritual practices we can cultivate is the discipline of taking our thoughts captive and submitting them to God.

Let's get practical. This means that we must actively and intentionally remind ourselves of what we know to be true of God. Remind yourself that he is mighty to save (Isa. 63:1). That he is "a God merciful and gracious, slow to anger, and abounding in steadfast love and faithfulness" (Ex. 34:6). Remind yourself that God is reigning over all things and that he is good in how he reigns. Remind yourself of what is true, honorable, just, pure, lovely, commendable, and excellent (Phil. 4:8). Because what we tell ourselves is an important part of how the battle for peace is won or lost.

Trusting the Lord is not always easy. It takes work. But the Lord is the only one worthy and able to hold all of our trust. And, as you and I intentionally submit our thoughts to the truth of who our God is, he will keep us in perfect peace.

Respond

Where have you seen the connection between trust and peace in your life? How important is it to have your mind stayed on God? What are some practical ways you can do that?

Request

Father, the trials, fears, worries, and sorrows of this world are real and can feel very overwhelming. I know that you can hold me through all of them. Help me to cling to you by fixing my mind on what you have told me in your word. And, Father, would the perfect peace that only you can give, the peace that passes all understanding, be mine in Christ today?

Be at Peace with All

Courtney Doctor

Read

> If possible, so far as it depends on you, live peaceably with all.
> (Rom. 12:18)

Reflect

You've probably heard the ditty that goes like this:

> To live above with the saints I love, well, that will be bliss
>   and glory.
> But to live below with the saints I know, well, that is another
>   story.

And don't we all know that to be true! We struggle to live peacefully with those around us—neighbors, coworkers, friends, and family. Disunity and strife are all around us, and they seem to affect believers and unbelievers alike. But is conflict inevitable?

We've already looked at two types of peace: peace *with* God and the peace *of* God. But, if you remember, the *shalom* we saw in the garden involved another type of peace: relational peace or peace with others.

We receive the peace that Jesus won for us on the cross. It's a free gift, given and received, not earned or deserved. But as a result of that free gift, we're called to live differently. We're called to be people who are characterized by peace: peaceful minds, peaceful homes, peaceful churches, peaceful relationships, and peaceful lives.

Because we've been reconciled, we pursue reconciliation with others. We ask for forgiveness and offer forgiveness (Col. 3:13). We consider others as more important than ourselves, look out for the interests of others (Phil. 2:3–4), and love others as we love ourselves (Mark 12:31). If we've been reconciled to the Father, the fruit of that reconciliation will show itself in our reconciliation with others.

Today's verse qualifies our pursuit of peace with the phrase, "so far as it depends on you." On one hand, this phrase challenges me. Am I pursuing peace as much as I possibly can? Am I forgiving, patient, humble, kind, counting the one with whom I struggle as more important than myself? Am I loving them, praying for them, seeking their good and not just mine? Do I move toward the people in my life with whom peace is difficult, or do I just shrug my shoulders and keep my distance?

On the other hand, this phrase comforts me by reminding me that this side of glory, not all relationships can or will be healed. The brokenness that disrupts our world impacts each one of us. We are all sinners, and we have all been sinned against—and this is true of every person with whom we struggle. As a result, some relationships may never experience the *shalom* we were created for. But the question remains, am I pursuing peace *as far as it depends on me*?

According to today's verse, peace is meant to permeate God's family. It's meant to draw us together over the things that would divide. We are meant to be reconciled with our brothers and sisters in Christ—in our churches, neighborhoods, and cities. Meaning, you and I are meant to experience *shalom* with those who vote differently, who live in a different part of town, and who don't look like us. We are meant to be pursuers of peace and extenders of *shalom* in every aspect of life.

The Prince of Peace has bought your peace. He freely gives it. But it's up to each of us, as far as it depends on us, to let that peace permeate our minds, our hearts, our homes, our churches, our cities, and our relationships. May the peace of Christ be yours today and every day.

Respond

In what ways are you both comforted and challenged by Paul's phrase "so far as it depends on you"? What barriers are most likely to prevent you from living in peace with others? Is there anyone specific with whom you need to pursue peace and reconciliation? What step could you take today to reach out to that person?

Request

Father, you have purchased my peace at the highest cost—the very life and death of your Son. Thank you that you have made a way for me. Help me to forgive others as I have been forgiven and to love others as I have been loved by you. Let me be an agent of peace in all the relationships you have given me.

Apple Breakfast Grain Bowl

Sharonda Cooper

This was my go-to recipe for the celebration brunch at the end of a year of Bible study. The ladies loved it! Just a few minutes in the kitchen before bedtime will fill your home with the aroma of apple-grain goodness.

Ingredients

- 2 cups whole grain (suggestion: 1 cup brown rice and 1 cup steel-cut oats)
- 2 peeled, chopped Granny Smith apples
- ½ cup chopped dried fruit (raisins, dates, dried cranberries, or a mixture)
- 5 cups water
- ¼ teaspoon cinnamon

Instructions

- Before going to bed, stir the ingredients together in a Crock-Pot. Turn the Crock-Pot on low heat and go to bed!

- In the morning, serve with a little honey or other sweetener and a splash of your favorite milk. (Optional toppings to add: chopped walnuts, butter, banana slices, blueberries)

Abide in Jesus

Melissa Kruger

Read

Abide in me, and I in you. As the branch cannot bear fruit by itself, unless it abides in the vine, neither can you, unless you abide in me. I am the vine; you are the branches. Whoever abides in me and I in him, he it is that bears much fruit, for apart from me you can do nothing. If anyone does not abide in me he is thrown away like a branch and withers; and the branches are gathered, thrown into the fire, and burned. (John 15:4–6)

Reflect

Every April, I spend a day preparing the soil in my garden. I pull up weeds, add compost, and start digging holes. By the time I'm done, I'm ready to plant tomatoes—Better Boy, Super Sweet Cherry, and my favorite, Cherokee Purple. Each plant begins small, but I space them a few feet apart because I know they'll grow much larger, bearing delicious fruit on their vines. As I dig, I'm dreaming about summertime salads and BLTs.

Eventually, April's bright hopes fade to gray with November's chill. One look at my garden, and I know it's time to discard the weary and worn vines. I roughly remove the tenderly planted stems and place them in a pile for the trash heap. The vines that used to be strong and vibrant now turn dry and dusty.

As I discard them, words from today's verses ring in my mind: "Apart from me you can do nothing." When a tree falls in my backyard, it can be fashioned into something else—furniture, a fort, a bridge, or a boat. But a vine removed from the soil simply withers away; it's unable to be used for anything else. My dry and dusty tomato vines remind me that life apart from Jesus is powerless and purposeless.

I hold this image in my mind each morning when I turn from the busyness that beckons to the pages of Scripture. I sit quietly before the word, taking in its nourishment, letting it feed my soul. There's so much to be done, but my tomato vines remind me of what's most important. Without Jesus, I'm not able to thrive. Without Jesus, I'm not able to survive. Apart from him, I can do *nothing*.

It may look to the watching world like we're doing something. We may be busy tending many things, appearing productive. Others may praise our efforts. However, our works without abiding will eventually display irritability, impatience, unkindness, harshness, and a lack of love. Weeds can grow in any garden, but they won't bear fruit.

To bear good fruit, we need time with Jesus. His word transforms us as the Spirit awakens our hearts and allows us to humbly serve others with love, joy, kindness, peace, and patience. Abiding in Jesus empowers our efforts so that good fruit beautifully adorns our good works.

Respond

Why is it important to abide in Jesus on a daily basis? What happens when we neglect time in the word or prayer? How does it impact our service to others?

Request

Dear Father, remind me that my love for others begins by abiding in Jesus. Keep me from a busyness that prevents me from spending daily time in the word and in prayer. By the power of your Spirit, let me walk in a manner worthy of the gospel, bearing fruit in every good work.

PATIENCE

Patience necessarily follows hope. For when it is grievous to be without the good you may desire, unless you sustain and comfort yourselves with patience, you must necessarily faint through despair. Hope then ever draws patience with it.

JOHN CALVIN[6]

Wait on the Lord

Megan Hill

Read

I waited patiently for the LORD;
    he inclined to me and heard my cry. (Ps. 40:1)

Reflect

What is patience? Often you know it when you *don't* see it. When you honk your horn in traffic, abandon your grocery cart in a huff in a crowded store, or snap at a coworker who walked in late to the meeting, you instantly recognize the *absence* of patience. We all know that grumbling and angry outbursts are signs that patience has left the building.

But if we want to cultivate patience in our hearts and lives, we need to move beyond acknowledging what it's *not* to begin understanding what it *is*. Scripture defines patience with several facets. Like a precious jewel, patience shines from multiple angles.

One facet of biblical patience is steadfastness, or endurance. When James holds up the Old Testament prophets as "an example of suffering and patience," he commends them as those "who remained steadfast" (James 5:10–11). Patience (or steadfastness) is faithfulness in difficult circumstances; it's continuing to follow Christ even when things are hard.

Another facet of patience is long-suffering. Paul calls the Ephesian Christians to godliness by urging them to put on "patience, bearing with one another in love, eager to maintain the unity of the spirit in the bond of peace" (Eph. 4:2–3). Long-suffering means we bear with difficult people. When Jesus told his disciples to forgive someone who sinned against them not just once or twice but "seventy-seven times" (Matt. 18:22), he was telling them to be patient.

A third biblical facet of patience is slowness to anger. James also writes, "Let every person be quick to hear, slow to speak, slow to anger; for the anger of man does not produce the righteousness of God" (James 1:19–20). It's important to note that the Bible doesn't forbid anger—sometimes anger is the righteous response to sin and injustice—but the Bible does forbid *hasty* anger. Patience takes the time to consider the situation and carefully act.

The final facet of patience overlaps the others. The Bible repeatedly describes patience as *waiting on the Lord*. In today's verse, the psalmist writes about a time when he was stuck. He was in a "miry bog" (v. 2) and didn't know how or when he'd get out. Maybe you can relate. Something as simple as being on hold with customer service or as hard as unwanted singleness can be a miry bog that makes you feel trapped. Our temptation in those moments is to be impatient, but the psalmist shows us a better way:

waiting on the Lord, trusting his goodness, and anticipating his care—no matter how long it takes.

Whatever our circumstances, it gives us courage to realize it's ultimately the Lord we're waiting on. Unlike the people in our lives, God is never late. He has good purposes for us even in our waiting, and when we wait on him, we can wait in hope.

Respond

Read Exodus 34:6–8. Make a list of the words and phrases God uses to describe himself to Moses. What words express God's patience? How does it comfort you to know that God is patient with you? How does God's patience encourage you to cultivate patience in your life?

Request

Dear Lord, I've been impatient too often. I've been sinfully anxious and focused on my circumstances, I've grumbled and complained, and I've treated others poorly. Forgive me. Please send your Spirit to cultivate patience in my heart. Make me steadfast, long-suffering, slow to anger, and ready to wait on you. Thank you for being merciful and gracious, slow to anger, and abounding in steadfast love.

Look in the Right Direction

Megan Hill

Read

> Let us run with endurance the race that is set before us, looking
> to Jesus, the founder and perfecter of our faith, who for the
> joy that was set before him endured the cross, despising the
> shame, and is seated at the right hand of the throne of God.
> (Heb. 12:1b–2)

Reflect

A few times in my life, I've experienced an MRI test. During an
MRI, you have to lie perfectly still on a table inside a tunnel-
shaped scanner. Once the medical technician begins capturing
the images, you can't sneeze, sniffle, or squirm. Of course, the
moment someone tells you that you can't move a muscle, every
inch of your skin begins to crawl. You may have been peacefully
resting before entering the tunnel, but suddenly you will go crazy
if you can't scratch that itch.

Trying to be patient is like having an MRI. As soon as you start thinking about how long-suffering and slow to anger you should be, every muscle in your body begins to twitch with impatience. The more you look at your circumstances and the more you tell yourself to relax, the more you just want to scream. The problem is that we can't be righteous in our own strength. Not one of us has the power to be patient on command.

In today's verses, the writer of Hebrews shows us that if we want to endure (remember, endurance is a biblical facet of patience) we have to focus our attention in the right place. If we look at all the things in our lives that are taking longer than we expected, we will quickly be tempted to give up. Whether it's the preschooler who insists on buttoning his own jacket or the employer who keeps choosing someone else for promotion or the illness that has baffled a dozen doctors, our circumstances defy our attempts to be patient. We can only endure when we look away from the trials and look toward Jesus.

Looking to Jesus as our example is the first way we grow in patience. Jesus faced incredibly difficult circumstances—including his shameful and painful death on the cross—but he endured. How? The writer to the Hebrews tells us that Jesus focused on "the joy that was set before him" (v. 2). When he was tempted to give up and give in to impatience, Jesus thought about how all of his people would one day be glorified and gathered with him in eternity, where he would be their acknowledged Lord and King. We can learn from Jesus's example and look ahead to heaven just like Jesus did.

The second way we grow in patience is by looking to Jesus for help. Christ was the only perfectly patient man, and in him we can become patient. On the cross, Christ broke sin's curse and grip on us and freed us to practice righteousness (see Rom. 6:5–14). When we call out to him for help, his Spirit enables us to resist temptation to impatience, to grow in love for others, to increase our trust in God's purposes, and to display patience in our lives (see Gal. 5:16–26). Jesus founded and perfected our faith (v. 2), and he helps us endure in our faith when we look to him.

Of course, we don't even have the power to look in the right place. Like Peter walking on the water (Matt. 14:22–33), we default to being overwhelmed by our circumstances. Even the ability to look to Jesus has to come from Jesus. Thankfully, he loves to give us this power. By sending his Spirit to dwell in us, Jesus has given us a divine helper who turns our eyes in the right direction—toward him.

Respond

Read Matthew 14:22–33. What were the circumstances of this story? What happened when Peter looked at the waves? Where should he have directed his focus? How does it encourage you to read that "Jesus . . . took hold of [Peter]" (v. 31)?

Request

Dear God, I can't be patient on my own. The more I think about being patient with _____ or patient in the middle of _____, the more impatient I get. Thank you for breaking sin's power over me and for creating a new heart in me. Please send your Spirit to turn my eyes to Jesus, the founder and perfecter of my faith.

Enroll in the School of Patience

Megan Hill

Read

Count it all joy, my brothers, when you meet trials of various kinds, for you know that the testing of your faith produces steadfastness. (James 1:2–3)

Reflect

I don't like to sweat. I don't like getting dirty. And I don't like bugs. It may surprise you, then, to know that every summer our family plants a vegetable garden. We haul (dirty) seedlings out to the (buggy) raised bed and we plant them with our (sweaty) hands. Over the spring and summer we get dirtier and buggier and sweatier as we water, weed, and prune. Why? There is nothing as wonderful as a homegrown tomato.

The promise of a ripe, red, juicy tomato makes me willing to do uncomfortable things. Likewise, it's only when we appreciate the value of patience that we will be eager to cultivate it in our lives.

Our verses today tell us that trials are the school of patience. We learn to endure in the faith by experiencing challenges to our faith. We learn to be long-suffering when we encounter people who sin against us. We learn to be slow to anger when our circumstances are not ideal. We learn to wait on the Lord when we don't get what we want when we want it. It's hardship—not ease—that produces steadfastness.

Knowing this, many of us would rather pass on cultivating patience. If it's going to require us to enroll in the school of difficulty (and James says it will), we'd rather play hooky. So, it's surprising that James encourages believers to "count it all joy" when God brings us into his classroom. James can tell us to rejoice in suffering because the goal is worth it. For James, becoming steadfast—trusting the Lord's goodness and continuing to follow Christ even when it's hard—is a precious result that makes trials worthwhile.

Scripture repeatedly affirms the lasting value of patience. It's one of God's attributes (Ex. 34:6), something God commands (Col. 3:12), a virtue God's people have always prized and practiced (Heb. 11:13), and a blessing to people around us (Phil. 3:1). James says the steadfast person is "blessed" and will "receive the crown of life" in eternity (James 1:12). Growing in patience is absolutely worth it.

Although you may not feel like you are learning patience right now, James writes about trials "of various kinds," reminding us that all kinds of circumstances can teach us patience. The ten-minute line at the drive-thru, the months of infertility, the years of estrangement from a sibling, and the lifetime of chronic illness are each tools in the hand of the Lord to allow us to practice steadfastness. And yesterday's lessons enable us to draw on increased faith as we encounter today's difficulties.

Day by day, the Lord is teaching you the unfading grace of patience. Count it all joy.

Respond

"Don't pray for patience! God just might give it to you!" we sometimes tell one another with a wink and a nudge. Have you ever felt that way? When? What does our fear of hardship tell us about how much we value the end result? Spend a few minutes reading the verses mentioned in today's devotional and meditating on the value of patience.

Request

Lord, I don't want to be patient. I know that the school of patience is filled with trials, and I'd like my life to be as easy as possible. I don't like to wait, and I don't like to bear with people who sin against me—and, if I'm honest, I don't really want opportunities to learn to do that. Please forgive me. Please send your Spirit to help me value what you value. Help me to count it all joy as I become more like my patient Savior, Jesus Christ.

Time Is Short

Megan Hill

Read

> You also, be patient. Establish your hearts, for the coming of the
> Lord is at hand. Do not grumble against one another, brothers,
> so that you may not be judged; behold, the Judge is standing
> at the door. (James 5:8–9)

Reflect

I regularly see a meme on social media that goes something like this:
"Adulting is saying, 'Next week will be less busy,' over and over until
you die." The joke is tinged with both humor and despair. Most
people over the age of eighteen can relate to looking forward to a
day when their calendar is clear and their to-do list is completely
checked off—only to see their anticipated free time evaporate as
new responsibilities appear on the horizon. And all the while, days
quickly turn into months and months turn into years. In the crazi-
ness of life, we can't help feeling that there is never enough time.

In today's verse, James tells us that we're right. Time *is* short, he says. Jesus's return is so close that it's "at hand." From the perspective of eternity, our days on earth are brief (Ps. 103:15–16), and Christ's coming is in the near future (Rev. 22:7). For believers, this is actually good news. Although the tasks of today and tomorrow and the next day may *feel* endless, they aren't. One day soon, Jesus will "descend from heaven with a cry of command," he will take us with him, and "we will always be with the Lord" (1 Thess. 4:16, 17). Be patient. This life is not forever. A better life is coming.

James also tells us that the shortness of time should have implications for how we relate to the people around us. Immediately after reminding us that we are running out of time, James commands, "Do not grumble against one another" (James 5:9). I don't know about you, but James's words make me squirm a bit. The Lord obviously knows that my greatest temptation when I'm short on time is to be short with other people.

But the shortness of time should lead us to do the opposite. *Because* we don't have much time, *because* Jesus is coming back, *because* we will all face the judgment of God, we ought to be slow to anger. When Christ returns, we want to be found loving others well. One of the ways we do that is to patiently bear with one another, humbly putting others' needs before our own. Why waste our limited time on impatience when we could use it to display the Spirit's fruit of patience?

Although James specifically mentions our relationships to other believers ("brothers and sisters"), our patient, nongrumbling conduct can also have evangelistic purposes in the lives of those who are not yet part of the family of God. The Lord is "patient toward you, not wishing that any should perish, but that all should reach repentance" (2 Pet. 3:9). When we are patient toward unbelievers—remembering that without Christ they face judgment and an eternity apart from God—we reflect the patience of our long-suffering God who doesn't delight in the destruction of sinners but who bears with them as long as he possibly can (Ezek. 33:11). Our patience can be a light that illuminates the Savior's love for a people walking in darkness.

Respond

Read Mark 10:17–22. What was Jesus doing when the man approached him? How might you act if someone interrupted you just as you were leaving the house or beginning a trip? How does Jesus respond? In what ways might our time and attention be a spiritual blessing to someone else?

Request

Thank you, Lord, for your patience toward me. Thank you also for the unbelievers you have placed in my life. Help me to be long-suffering with them, remembering that time is short. Give me compassion for their undying souls. Please use my patience to teach others about your patience and to point them to Jesus.

Farmstand Blueberry Cobbler

Lydia Brownback

When a quick summer dessert is called for, quarts of just-picked blueberries are readily available at just about every roadside farmstand on the outskirts of most villages in Central New York. When the summer supply is plentiful, this cobbler makes a weekly appearance at our family table.

Serves 4-6
Preheat oven to 375 degrees

Ingredients

- 6 tablespoons butter
- 1 cup flour
- 2 teaspoons baking powder
- ½ teaspoon salt
- ½ teaspoon nutmeg
- 1 cup sugar
- ⅔ cup milk
- 2 cups fresh blueberries

Instructions

- In 2-quart baking dish or 8 x 8 baking pan, melt butter.

- In a large bowl, whisk flour, baking powder, salt, and nutmeg; then stir in sugar until just combined. Stir in milk.

- Pour the batter over the melted butter. Do not stir.

- Pour the berries into the center. Do not stir.

- Bake 35 minutes or until golden.

- Serve with vanilla ice cream or whipped cream.

KINDNESS

*If there is one virtue which most commends Christians,
it is that of kindness. . . . Imitate Christ in your loving
spirits: speak kindly, act kindly, and do kindly, that
men may say of you, "He has been with Jesus."*

CHARLES SPURGEON[7]

Kindness Might Surprise You

Winfree Brisley

Read

Be kind to one another, tenderhearted, forgiving one another, as God in Christ forgave you. (Eph. 4:32)

Reflect

We were shopping a high-end consignment sale—three women on a mission to find designer clothes at affordable prices. My friend popped out of the fitting room beaming about the dress she had on. The design was unique, the colors were vibrant, and the price was right. There was only one problem—it was hideous! As I tried to beat around the bush, unsure whether to tell her the truth, our other friend walked up and politely, but firmly, advised that the dress was a no-go. We all still laugh about that dress!

At the time, I probably thought I was being kind by not bursting my friend's bubble, but the truth is, I was just being nice—agreeable and pleasant. The friend who told the truth was kind.

You see, although we tend to use *nice* and *kind* as synonyms, they're actually different.

Kindness in the Bible has two facets: it meets a need, and it avoids harshness. Biblical kindness involves being useful, offering service that is well-fitted for a situation, and doing so in a gracious manner. It means doing good to others, freely and gladly.

Notice how Paul talks about kindness in today's verse. He tells the Ephesians to be "tenderhearted" and to forgive each other as they have been forgiven in Christ. Here we see kindness applied to relationships. It's easy to be nice to people who are nice to us. But when others sin against us and we respond with tenderness and forgiveness, we demonstrate kindness.

Kindness also relates to how we care for others practically. Paul encourages the Philippian church, "It was kind of you to share my trouble" (Phil. 4:14). The surrounding verses indicate that Paul is thanking them for a financial gift, but the way he describes their help is telling. They didn't just send money—they *shared his trouble*. We can give away a lot of money without truly extending kindness. The Philippians gave of their resources to meet Paul's needs *and* sympathized with him in his trouble.

It's probably not much of a stretch for us to understand the kindness in Paul's examples. Being tenderhearted, forgiving, and sharing troubles—these all make sense to us as kindness. But biblical kindness sometimes expresses itself in unexpected ways.

In Psalm 141, David says, "Let a righteous man strike me—it is a kindness; let him rebuke me—it is oil for my head" (v. 5). Does David's definition of kindness differ from Paul's? Not at all! David is saying that it would be kind for a godly man to point out his sin. Because we can be blind to our sin, we sometimes need others to help us see it. David compares a rebuke to oil poured on his head, a sign of honor. To say hard things, to share the truth of Scripture, and even to do so directly, is not the same as being harsh (though we must take care to speak graciously). We do good to others, indeed, we show kindness, when we tell the truth—whether it's about sin issues or ugly dresses.

Kindness can look different depending on the situation. So how can we know what it means to be kind moment-to-moment as we go about our days? We look to our God who is "kind in all his works" (Ps. 145:17), asking the Holy Spirit to make us more like him.

Respond

Read Ruth 1:1–18. What are some of the ways Naomi and Ruth display kindness to each other? How does Naomi believe the Lord will treat her daughters-in-law in the midst of their suffering (v. 8)? How have you experienced the Lord's kindness in your own times of suffering and need?

Request

Father, you are kind in all your works, but I often fall short. Forgive me for ignoring the needs of others. Forgive me for being harsh. By the work of your Holy Spirit, please give me a heart that is tender, hands that are ready to serve, and a mouth that graciously speaks the truth. Thank you for always dealing kindly with me.

Jesus Frees You to Be Kind

Winfree Brisley

Read

Come to me, all who labor and are heavy laden, and I will give you rest. Take my yoke upon you, and learn from me, for I am gentle and lowly in heart, and you will find rest for your souls. For my yoke is easy, and my burden is light. (Matt. 11:28–30)

Reflect

Early in our marriage, my husband and I planned a visit to the college town where we met. We decided to splurge and stay at a beautiful historic inn near campus. When we checked in, we were shocked to find that our large bill was already paid. Years later, we learned that my husband's uncle was responsible. As a fellow alumnus, he understood both the significance and the cost of staying at the inn. What kindness on his part—and what a relief for us! Because he bore the cost, we were free to enjoy our stay without worry.

In today's verses, Jesus displays a similar, though much more profound, kindness. Jesus uses the imagery of a yoke—a beam of wood laid across the backs of animals to enable them to pull a plow or cart—in other words, a heavy load. And he says that he will take our heavy yoke and give us his easy one (v. 30). Interestingly, the Greek word translated there as "easy" is the same word we find elsewhere in the New Testament translated as "kind."

Indeed, it's not hard to see kindness in the exchange Jesus describes. He sees our weariness; he knows the burdens we carry; he understands our need for rest and tenderly offers us an easier load. But why are we so weary in the first place, and how can Jesus lighten our burden?

If we try to name the things that weigh us down, we might talk about anxiety and depression, financial hardships, strained relationships, unfulfilled desires, and so much more. Those things are real, and Jesus cares about them. But there's an even deeper weight we carry—the burden of our sin.

Just try being kind for one day. Kind to your roommate. Kind to your husband. Kind to your boss. Kind to your kids. Kind to your nosy neighbor. Kind with your words—all of them. Kind in your thoughts—all of them. You get the idea. We can't do it!

Perfection is a heavy yoke to bear, and no matter how much we labor, we won't achieve it in our own strength. That's why Jesus offers us his perfection. He lived the perfect life that we couldn't, keeping every aspect of God's law. He took our sin—all of it—and bore the punishment for it on the cross. He died the death we deserve so that our debt is paid.

Jesus frees us from the weight and burden of our sin, but not so we can throw off the yoke and do whatever we want.

No, remember that this is an exchange—our heavy yoke for his easy one. Now that we are no longer slaves to our sin, we are free to obey God. We still live under God's law, but in Christ, his commandments are not burdensome (1 John 5:3). When we take on the yoke of Christ, we are transformed from slaves to sin to laborers in God's kingdom.

So we can be kind. We can meet the needs of others even when it costs us, knowing that our deepest needs are met in Christ. We can serve until we are tired, knowing that Jesus gives us rest for our souls. We can do good to others without expectation of return because we know that the Lord withholds no good thing from us (Ps. 84:11). In his kindness, God has met our greatest need in Jesus Christ, freeing us to show kindness to others.

Respond

Read Ephesians 2:4–10. How has God shown us kindness in Christ Jesus? Why is it important to understand that we are not saved *by* our good works, but we are saved *for* good works (vv. 9–10)? How does this difference encourage you as you seek to grow in kindness?

Request

Dear Lord, thank you that salvation is not dependent on my works, but on yours. I can't even be kind for one day, let alone keep all of your commandments perfectly. Thank you for taking the burden of my sin and giving me new life in Christ. Help me to be kind to others, not because I have to in order to earn your favor, but because I can through the power of your Holy Spirit working in me.

Put Off and Put On

Winfree Brisley

Read

Put on then, as God's chosen ones, holy and beloved, compassionate hearts, kindness, humility, meekness, and patience. (Col. 3:12)

Reflect

I love decorating my home with fresh flowers—unfortunately I have a brown thumb. The only flower I've successfully grown is the hydrangea. Thankfully, it's one of my favorites! And in the South where I live, they grow with little fuss. For my bushes to produce bountiful blooms, I only have to do one thing: deadhead them. Removing dead blooms preserves the plant's energy and encourages new blooms.

In Colossians 3, Paul uses a similar metaphor of putting off and putting on clothing to describe the changes that should take place in us as we are transformed into the image of Christ. In today's verse, he gives a list of characteristics that we should "put on," including kindness. We know that kindness is a fruit of the Spirit, and ultimately it's his work in us that produces kindness. But Paul's wording also suggests that we have an active role to play.

Paul says in verse 5, "Put to death therefore what is earthly in you." Just as I cut off old, dead blooms from my hydrangeas to prepare them for new growth, we need to spiritually "put off" (v. 9) our old, dead life of sin and divert our energy toward putting on the characteristics of godliness.

So what sin might we need to put off in order to cultivate kindness? Paul includes a long list of sins that we should put to death, but let's consider three that particularly inhibit kindness: covetousness, anger, and slander.

Covetousness means having a greedy desire for more things or for things that belong to someone else. Whereas kindness looks to meet the needs of others, covetousness looks to fulfill our own desires. If we have a covetous spirit, we will hold tightly to what we have and focus our energy on getting more.

We may become angry when we feel disrespected, when our expectations aren't met, or when we have been wronged. Maybe anger flares up when our child disobeys or our coworker doesn't pull her weight. Kindness is tender toward others, but anger can harden us against them. And it often overflows in harshness.

While kindness uses words to do good to others, slander means talking about someone in a way that injures her good name. We might not be so bold as to invent damaging information about someone, but have we ever embellished the truth to make it sound worse? Have we shared unflattering details about another woman's life under the guise of a prayer request?

Clipping off dead hydrangea blooms is pretty easy, but putting off sin feels a bit more complicated, right? This is where Paul's clothing analogy might be more helpful than my gardening one. If we take off a dirty shirt, we replace it with a clean one. Similarly, when we seek to put off sin, we need to replace it with some aspect of godliness.

Paul tells us, "Set your minds on things that are above, not on things that are on earth" (Col. 3:2). In other words, if we want to put off covetousness, anger, and slander, one of the best things we can do is set our minds on kindness. Meditate on the kindness of God, and ask him to bear a bountiful harvest in you by the work of his Spirit.

Respond

Read Hosea 11:4. This verse describes God's fatherly care for his children, Israel. What do you learn about God's kindness from Hosea's imagery? How does it encourage you to know that this is how God cares for you?

Request

Dear Father, I want to grow in kindness. Please work in my heart to root out sins like coveting, anger, and slander, and replace them with seeds of kindness. As your Spirit works in my heart, help me to actively set my mind on things above, things like your kindness and tender care for me.

Kindness Is Not Random

Winfree Brisley

Read

Thus says the LORD of hosts, Render true judgments, show kindness and mercy to one another. (Zech. 7:9)

Reflect

When I was in high school, I played tennis—though not very well. One of my challenges was getting enough practice in the offseason. I would sometimes drive over to the courts and hit against a practice wall, but balls ricocheting at close range don't quite simulate a real match. To really practice tennis, you need another person.

Similarly, kindness is one fruit of the Spirit that we can't practice in isolation. We might experience peace in our own hearts and minds or exercise self-control when we're alone, but we demonstrate kindness in relationship. As today's verse illustrates, kindness isn't something we show to ourselves; it's something we show to one another.

Being kind has become a popular virtue in our culture. As I write today on February 17, it just so happens to be National Random Acts of Kindness Day. Perhaps you've paid for the coffee of the person behind you in line or left a gift card at the gas pump as a way of participating in one of these kindness initiatives. Random acts of kindness can be fun, and there's nothing wrong with this sort of generosity.

But in the Bible, kindness is not bestowed randomly—it's intentional and specific. Think back to Paul's and David's examples from day 19 of believers being kind to one another. These weren't strangers. They were members of the same congregation. And Jesus teaches in Luke 6:35: "Love your enemies, and do good, and lend, expecting nothing in return, and your reward will be great, and you will be sons of the Most High, for he is kind to the ungrateful and the evil."

Jesus tells us to be kind to some very specific people: our enemies. Why? So that we will be like our Father in heaven who is kind to the ungrateful and the evil. Our culture's response to enemies, the ungrateful, and the evil is to cancel them, to destroy their reputations online, to cut them off from relationship. Cultural kindness is either random or reserved for the worthy—people we agree with, people who affirm us, people we deem good.

But if we as believers in Christ are kind to our enemies, kind to the ungrateful, and kind to the evil, others will see a difference. Maybe it's how we interact with the ungrateful family member who criticizes us at every turn. Maybe it's how we respond to the dishonest boss who takes credit for our ideas. Maybe it's how we serve the neighbor turned nemesis who lets her dog destroy our yard. When we show kindness in specific ways to people who are hard to love, we reflect the kindness of God. And his kindness has a wonderfully specific purpose—to lead sinners to repentance (Rom. 2:4).

If you're like me, you might be wishing you could go back to thinking of kindness as paying for a stranger's coffee. Biblical kindness sounds hard! That's why we have to remember that kindness requires relationship. We demonstrate kindness in our relationships with others—but we grow in kindness through our relationship with Christ. We look to the Holy Spirit's work in us to bear the fruit of kindness, and we pray that he would work in the hearts of our enemies, the ungrateful, and the evil to bring them to repentance.

Respond

Read 2 Samuel 9:1–13. How does David intentionally and specifically pursue kindness? Why is it significant that David wants to show kindness to someone from the house of Saul? How does David's kindness to Mephibosheth reflect God's kindness to us?

Request

Dear Lord, thank you that when I was your enemy, you showed me kindness by sending your Son to die for me. Thank you that your kindness has led me to repentance and into relationship with you. Through the work of your Spirit, help me show kindness, especially to someone who is hard to love, like _____. Please work in _____'s heart. Show her your kindness and bring her to repentance.

Raspberry Sorbet
Winfree Brisley

My husband's aunt is a wonderful cook, and she has a talent for finding delicious recipes that are shockingly easy. This raspberry sorbet is a prime example. Keep a bag of raspberries in your freezer, and you can have a delightful, refreshing dessert ready in no time, anytime you need it!

Serves 4

Ingredients

- ¼ cup water
- ¼ cup plus 1 tablespoon sugar
- 1 bag (12 ounces) frozen raspberries (or freeze 3 cups fresh raspberries)

Instructions

- Whisk together the water and ¼ cup of sugar until the sugar dissolves.

- Pulse the raspberries in a food processor until coarsely chopped. While the food processor is still running, pour in the sugar-water. Continue to pulse until the mixture is smooth.

- Transfer the raspberry mixture to an airtight container and freeze it until firm (at least 30 minutes).

GOODNESS

God is goodness itself, in whom all goodness is involved.
If therefore we love other things for the goodness which
we see in them, why do we not love God, in whom
is all goodness? All other things are but sparks of that
fire, and drops of that sea. If you see any good in the
creature, remember there is much more in the Creator.

RICHARD SIBBES[8]

Show Us Your Goodness

Lindsey Carlson

Read

I believe that I shall look upon the goodness of the LORD
in the land of the living! (Ps. 27:13)

Reflect

How can imperfect people like you and me arrive at a solid definition of goodness when we can't even agree on which books, movies, sports teams, or restaurants are good? Can goodness be objectively observed and shared with others?

When we use the word *good*, we are usually referring to something that is pleasing, desirable, or beneficial. But when the Bible uses the word *good*, it attests to what is pleasing, desirable, and good *to God*. When the psalmist declares with confidence, "I believe that I shall look upon the goodness of the LORD in the land of the living" in Psalm 27:13, he knows that in this broken world, remnants of God's goodness remain.

God is the source of all good; he who created the heavens and the earth and spoke light into darkness looked on his own creation and saw that it was good (Gen. 1:4). He brought forth the land and the seas, the grass, seed, and trees yielding fruit after their own kind (Gen. 1:11–12), the day ruling over the night (Gen. 1:18), and every living thing (Gen. 1:21) and saw that it was good. Then God created mankind. And he called us "very good" (Gen. 1:31). All goodness flows from him and through him.

God shares his goodness with mankind. He created us in his own image and gave us dominion over the earth and all that is in it. As image bearers, we are born into his good world filled with his good gifts, so that we might enjoy the goodness of God both now and forevermore—in the land of the living and forever in eternity with him.

When we ask God to show us his goodness, we're often looking for him to provide goods and services by answering our request with a good job opportunity, a good paycheck, or a good gift we can hold in our hands. But God displays his goodness to his people for a purpose grander than our satisfaction or enjoyment. Consider when Moses wearily leads rebellious Israel through the wilderness and cries out in desperation to God. As he pleads to see God's glory that he might be sustained, God answers, "I will make all my goodness pass before you and will proclaim before you my name 'The LORD'" (Ex. 33:19). God displays his goodness in order to reveal his glory to his children so we would be moved to give thanks and rejoice in him.

God's ultimate display of goodness is found in the provision of Christ, who declared his perfect love by dying to save sinners. Since we cannot earn God's forgiveness, he sent his Son so that

Christ's goodness might cover our sins. Goodness can be summarized as Christ's love in action. The Spirit gives us the fruit of goodness so we can share Christ's love with others.

Through the gift of the Holy Spirit, Christ's followers can go out and do good (Acts 10:38), displaying the spiritual fruit of goodness (Gal. 5:22), and proclaiming the good news of the kingdom of God (Luke 8:1) for the common good (1 Cor. 12:7) of those he calls to himself. God's people experience the goodness of God and then share it with the world! By bearing the fruit of goodness, we magnify God as the source and strength of all that is desirable and beneficial.

Respond

Read Psalm 31:19–22. What words does the psalmist use to describe God's goodness to those who fear him? How does God protect his people? What does he promise to display to them? Think of a difficult season in your life. Ask the Holy Spirit to help you discern ways God was present with you and to think of specific ways he displayed his goodness.

Request

Lord, I confess that I'm tempted to look for displays of your goodness apart from you. I want blessings and rewards that have little to do with your name or your glory. Forgive and cleanse my heart, Lord, through Christ Jesus. Draw me to your word where I might gaze upon your beauty and goodness and rest in your presence. Teach me to be satisfied not by worldly riches, but by everything you declare is good, right, and perfectly pleasing to you. Help me to seek your goodness that I might extend your good to the world you created.

Goodness Requires Practice

Lindsey Carlson

Read

Why do you ask me about what is good? There is only one who is good. (Matt. 19:17)

Reflect

As a child learning to play the piano, I memorized the phrase "Every Good Boy Does Fine." This simple technique helped me remember the names of the notes on the treble staff. That's about all it did for me, because even though I plucked the proper keys as a kindergartner, my playing didn't sound pretty. Developing skill and proficiency that actually sounded good and beautiful took time.

In a similar way, it takes time to grow in our ability to bear the fruit of goodness. We must do more than memorize the names of the fruit. We must also study Christ's goodness and practice extending it to others through our attitudes and actions. And we must pray and wait patiently for God to cultivate and nourish the growing fruit.

We see the fruit of goodness repeatedly throughout the life of Christ. In Matthew 19:16, Jesus encountered a rich young man who knelt and asked him, "Teacher, what good deed must I do to have eternal life?" Jesus offered no quick and easy answers. He didn't praise the man's good track record of law-abiding behavior or say he was doing fine. Instead Jesus reminded the man, "No one is good except God alone" (Mark 10:18). Goodness points others directly to God as the source of all good.

Jesus looked at the rich man, "loved him, and said to him, 'You lack one thing: go, sell all that you have and give to the poor, and you will have treasure in heaven; and come, follow me" (Mark 10:21). By commending the practice of sacrificial living and discipleship, Jesus pointed the rich man to a better treasure: eternal riches in heaven, which are good to store up.

Goodness also confronts sin and wickedness, for the good of others. When Jesus entered the temple, overturned the tables, and drove out the moneychangers who'd turned his house into a den of robbers (Matt. 21:11–13), we are quick to note his anger. But while his wrath didn't feel great to the moneychangers, Jesus's actions were for the good of others; he was protecting the purity of God's holy temple. Goodness can be demonstrated by standing up for what is good and true.

Christ encourages our pursuit of goodness. When Mary and Martha welcomed Jesus into their house for a meal (Luke 10:42), Mary spent the afternoon sitting at the Lord's feet, enthralled by his teaching. In response, she later knelt before him and anointed his feet (John 12:1–3). And Jesus praised Mary for choosing "the good portion," which he promised would "not be taken away from her" (Luke 10:42). Christ helps his people lay hold of lasting goodness.

Christ fills our lives with good. Romans 8:28 says, "We know that for those who love God all things work together for good." Just as the boy Jesus had to learn and grow in favor with God and man (Luke 2:52), we must watch and learn and grow too. We shouldn't be surprised when it takes time for us to develop skill and proficiency in displaying God's goodness. When we fix our eyes on Christ and walk by the Holy Spirit, he will bring forth fruit. As the gospel melody flows through our lives, the notes of goodness will sing a joyful song of salvation that will move listeners to delight in Christ.

Respond

Read Isaiah 63:7. Notice the way remembering the Lord's mercy is a decision: "I will recount the steadfast love of the LORD . . . and the great goodness . . . of his steadfast love." Are you ever tempted to fix your mind on trials and trouble and to forget the goodness of God? How might you remember and recount his goodness in times like these? How might you prioritize the good portion?

Request

Lord, apart from you I have no good. Teach me to follow Jesus and to do good to others. Help me to recognize when others are bound in sin or transgression and to speak truthfully for their good. Help me to provide them with the good news of salvation in a way that brings goodness and light to their lives. Make me, in the words of Jeremiah, "radiant over the goodness of the LORD" so that my life would be like a watered garden providing your good and living water to all who thirst.

Goodness Looks Good on You

Lindsey Carlson

Read

Beloved, do not imitate evil but imitate good. Whoever does good is from God; whoever does evil has not seen God. Demetrius has received a good testimony from everyone, and from the truth itself. We also add our testimony, and you know that our testimony is true. (3 John 11–12)

Reflect

Before I came to a saving faith in Christ, God gave me a few good Christian friends. And while they may not have known one another, they had some things in common. They followed the rules. They didn't lie, cheat, or steal. Their words blessed and did not curse. They were kind and gentle with others. And they were unashamed to speak publicly of their faith in Christ.

They also shared the same unflattering nickname among our peers at school and at church. Each girl was called a "goody-goody" because of what some perceived as annoyingly good behavior and excessive politeness. Friends and classmates doubted their sincerity.

These girls weren't insincere; they were mature followers of Christ whose good fruit served as a true testimony to the transformative work of salvation and sanctification. They were credible witnesses to the fact that they believed the promises of God.

The fruit of goodness is important in a believer's life because it tells a story of transformation; apart from the Spirit, the desire to turn away from evil and toward God's good is unusual. But when we've tasted and seen that God is good, we want to grow in godliness in order to point humanity to the presence of God, whose goodness is evident in all his creation (Gen. 1:31). Just like the leper whom Jesus healed or the blind whose sight was restored, our changed lives draw attention and invite countless opportunities to boast in the resurrected power of Christ.

In the Old Testament, God repeatedly spoke of his promised good to Abraham, Isaac, Jacob, Moses, and Joshua. Throughout Israel's days of slavery, of waiting and wandering, of conquering and rebuilding, God's good promises sustained the faith of his people as they shared them from generation to generation. By passing along the same good news and living lives that testify to the same good promises, the fruit of goodness blossoms in our own hearts, before it reproduces throughout the family of God.

Today, through Christ's death and resurrection, we are witnesses to God's goodness as we lead lives of sincerity. We love God and others. We flee sin. We cling to what is good. Our words and actions demonstrate that we are indeed a new creation, transformed by the Father's love. And when we join our voices together with all the saints, our stories become "a testimony to all the nations" (Matt. 9:35; 24:14) that God utilizes to transform our friends and family members, our cities and villages, as the gospel goes forth throughout the whole world.

The fruit of goodness should not be contained or hidden. We must speak of what we love. In Psalm 78, the psalmist proclaims that Israel will declare all the glorious deeds of the Lord to the coming generation (vv. 3–4). It is good to sing praises to him, to "tell of all his wondrous works" (1 Chron. 16:9), and to "tell of his salvation from day to day" (1 Chron. 16:23)!

The fruit of goodness isn't intended to make you look good; it's meant to make God look good. Don't be a goody-goody. Be a sincere follower of Jesus who looks upon the goodness of God and lets your light shine before others "so that they may see your good works and give glory to your Father who is in heaven" (Matt. 5:16).

Respond

Read Matthew 5:13–15 and Luke 8:16–18. Have you ever been tempted to keep God's goodness to yourself because you fear sounding insincere or like a goody-goody? How is the Spirit challenging you to rise and declare God's goodness to others? How might you provide a sincere, good testimony to your family members, your neighbors, or your community?

Request

Lord, help me to boldly proclaim your goodness to my friends, my family, and to the coming generations. May I tell of your might and the wonders you have done. By the light of your Spirit, make known your deeds in my life and among your people so that I will give thanks to you. You are my Lord; I have no good apart from you. For you, O Lord, are good and forgiving, abounding in steadfast love to all who call upon you.

Share the Goodness!

Lindsey Carlson

Read

When the goodness and loving kindness of God our Savior appeared, he saved us, not because of works done by us in righteousness, but according to his own mercy. (Titus 3:4)

Reflect

Rolling over in the darkness under the warmth of my covers, I reached to silence my phone's alarm. On the screen was an unanswered text message: "You good?"

I wasn't. Sick in bed with the flu, my lingering fever indicated I was still contagious. No matter how much I wanted to be good enough to get up out of the bed in that moment, there was nothing I could do to heal myself. Similarly, sin and brokenness plague our hearts and prevent us from recognizing God's merciful goodness.

Titus 3:4 assures believers that "when the goodness and loving kindness of God our Savior appeared," Christ saved us. He was good to us. He healed us when we were undeserving. As recipients of God's good, we should see and appreciate each gift of grace as evidence of God's goodness and want to share them with others.

It's not always easy to want to share God's goodness with others. When a stranger cuts me off in traffic and then moments later wants me to let him merge in front of me, I'm not naturally inclined to oblige. I'd rather honk my horn and give him a look that says, "No way."

Thankfully, I'm not left to my own inclinations. In moments of selfishness, the Spirit humbles and convicts me. God has been so good to me. Surely I can pardon an angry driver. So instead I smile, wave, and let him over. Opportunities to provide others with good exist around every corner.

Even more than showing goodness to a stranger on the road, I need the Spirit's help in my closest relationships. It isn't always easy to provide good to my neighbors, my friends, or even to my family. On nights I know it would be good to read Scripture at the dinner table with my children or to linger in prayer with my husband, I'm tempted to be selfish. I'd rather rush through dinner and on to dishes when I'm tired. But my lack of desire to do good to others is like that fever reminding me I can't make myself better. I have a continual need for Christ's mercy. And over time, his goodness changes us.

Because goodness is ours through Christ, we seek the good of others. Our time, energy, finances, gifts, and talents and our labors are all tools God mercifully grants to allow us to share his goodness with others. The Spirit compels us as believers to devote ourselves to good works that are excellent and profitable for others (Titus 3:7–9) and then fills us with the fruit of goodness so we might devotedly attend to good works that serve our friends, our coworkers, our spouse, or our children. The Spirit helps us prioritize the good of the moment for the sake of eternity.

Respond

Read Psalm 145:1–9. How does David respond to God as he ponders his unsearchable greatness? Who does he say will "commend" God's works to another and pour forth the fame of his abundant goodness? Because the Lord is good to all, and his mercy is over all he has made, you are called to tell of his wondrous works. Who might you tell of his goodness today?

Request

Thank you, Lord, for your great goodness and beauty. Thank you that my life abounds with good because you are good to sinners. As you fill me with the fruit of goodness, enable me to abound with the goodness and loving kindness of the Savior, that others might taste the goodness of the word of God and the powers of the age to come.

Suffering Leads to Fruitfulness

Melissa Kruger

Read

Blessed is the man who trusts in the LORD,
  whose trust is the LORD.
He is like a tree planted by water,
  that sends out its roots by the stream,
and does not fear when heat comes,
  for its leaves remain green,
and is not anxious in the year of drought,
  for it does not cease to bear fruit. (Jer. 17:7–8)

Reflect

A few weeks ago, my mom called with news I didn't want to hear. Her cancer had returned, and this time it was stage IV. In some ways, I wasn't surprised by the news. She'd been losing weight, experiencing pain in her bones, and feeling exhausted. At the same time, the news hit me like a ton of bricks. I got off the phone, made a cup of tea, and sat down at my kitchen table and cried.

I know what cancer means. It means scans and treatments and doctor visits. It means waiting for one result and then another, and then more waiting. It's painful, unpredictable, and scary. And when it's stage IV, it's treatable but not curable. It's not going away.

How do we bear fruit in the difficult seasons of life? When the heat and drought threaten to consume, is it even possible? In today's verses, the prophet Jeremiah guides us to hope by telling us about a tree. When heat leads to drought, and barrenness envelopes the landscape, somehow the tree remains vibrant and green. How is this possible?

The tree is planted by water.

In the midst of the drought, the tree has enough. Its roots have traveled underground, finding a path to a source that's independent of outward circumstances. When there's no rain, there's still nourishment. When there's drought, there's still fruit.

Suffering comes in a variety of forms: loss, pain, longing, illness, death. We search for words to describe the barrenness and brokenness, but whatever the suffering, we all experience a deep thirst, a longing for something to satisfy our souls. We're parched. Exhausted. Depleted. Weary. We need a stream from which to drink.

In the midst of Israel's thirst in the desert wilderness, they cried out to Moses. He struck the rock at Horeb and out poured miraculous refreshment. Over a thousand years later, Jesus stood up and offered, "If anyone thirsts, let him come to me and drink" (John 7:37). He's the everlasting spring, providing us miraculous refreshment in the scorched places of our lives.

When all else is barren, we begin to understand the true source of our fruitfulness. As Puritan Thomas Lye explained, "When we have no bread to eat, or water to drink, but only afflictions and astonishments, this is a time . . . for trusting. An Almighty God can work without means. God often brings his people into such a condition that they do not know what to do. *He does this that they might know what he can do.*"[9]

Blessed is the person who trusts in the Lord. Because of Christ, we need not be anxious when outer comforts are removed. We have an available, eternal stream from which to drink. We trust. God makes a way in the wilderness.

Respond

What difficult circumstance are you facing today? What truth about God can you meditate on throughout the day to help you trust in him?

Request

Lord, in my suffering, let me trust you. You are good. You are powerful. You are unchanging. You reign over all things. When I can't understand what to do, let me turn in dependence to you. Oh, Lord, in my barrenness, let me bear fruit.

Summer Fruit Cobbler
Melissa Kruger

We enjoy this cobbler every summer, especially when my blackberry bush and plum tree are overflowing with fresh fruit. It's perfect warm from the oven with a scoop of vanilla ice cream on top!

Ingredients
- 2 sticks butter
- 1½ cups brown sugar
- 3 cups oats
- 4–5 cups blueberries (I also use plums or blackberries or a mix of both)
- ¼ cup heavy cream
- ½ cup self-rising flour

- Preheat oven to 325 degrees and grease an oval 2.5-quart baking dish. Let butter come to room temperature. Cream brown sugar and butter together using a mixer. Stir in oatmeal by hand.

Instructions
- Spread one-third of the oat mixture in the baking dish, then half the berries, then another third of the oat mixture, then the remaining berries.

- Take the remaining third of the oat mixture and add cream and self-rising flour.* Layer this mixture over the berries to form a yummy crust. Bake for 35 minutes or until mixture is bubbling and brown on top.

*If you want to keep this recipe gluten-free, omit this step and just cover the cobbler with the remaining third of the oatmeal mixture.

FAITHFULNESS

*Sometimes when we read the words of those who have
been more than conquers, we feel almost despondent. I feel
that I shall never be like that. But they won through step
by step, by little bits of wills, little denials of self, little
inward victories, by faithfulness in very little things. They
became what they are. No one sees these hidden steps.
They only see the accomplishment, but even so, those
small steps were taken. There is no sudden triumph, no
spiritual maturity. That is the work of the moment.*

AMY CARMICHAEL[10]

Take Small Steps toward God

Blair Linne

Read

Let us hold fast the confession of our hope without wavering,
for he who promised is faithful. (Heb. 10:23)

Reflect

What is faithfulness? The Latin word for faith is *fide*. *Fide* is where
we get the word *fidelity*, which means "faithfulness." Fidelity to
a sport is faithfulness to the team. Parental fidelity is faithfulness
to one's offspring. Marital fidelity is faithfulness to a spouse.
Christian fidelity is faithfulness to God.

God has made a covenant with his people, promising to rescue
them from death. As Christians, we have received the Father's saving grace by the Spirit, through Jesus, by faith. Faith is essential
for our new birth. But faith is not a one-and-done. Christ's work
in us doesn't produce merely a profession of faith; it also produces
a heart that pursues faithfulness. Faithfulness is our continued
loyalty to our God and his gracious covenant.

As our verse for today explains, God's faithfulness to us is the bedrock for our faithfulness to God. As we behold him, we will be like him, the epitome of faithfulness. Only through considering his faithfulness do we mature into a faith that is proven genuine. Moment by moment as we follow Jesus, cast off our sin, and take up our new nature, we grow in faithfulness.

Faithfulness grows when, despite resistance, we take the step to trust in the object of our faith: Jesus. He told us that in this world we would face trouble. The trials help us mature as we hide ourselves in the faithful one who overcame the world. Faithfulness isn't gritting our teeth and mustering up self-determination. If we take Jesus out of the picture, we may have grit, but we don't have faithfulness. He allows us to take steps and eventually run with endurance despite hardship, "looking to Jesus, the founder and perfecter of our faith" (Heb. 12:2).

Spirit-produced faithfulness looks like fighting to prioritize time in the word during a busy season. It looks like showing up for church when you are exhausted from getting the kids ready and tempted to give up and stay home. Faithfulness looks like repenting of sin that no one else knows about or may recognize because you desire to honor God in private more than impress men in public. Faithfulness is clinging to a faithful God who is the same yesterday, today, and forever by choosing to trust in his covenant and take a step toward him right now.

Respond

Frequently in Hebrew poetry we find God's faithfulness linked to his steadfast love. Read Psalms 25:10; 36:5; 57:3; 108:4; and Lamentations 3:22–23. The word for steadfast love in these passages is *hesed*. *Hesed* is God's covenant-keeping love, a promise based on his character, not our own. In what ways have you experienced God's faithfulness?

Request

God, I praise you. You are faithful. I am so often unfaithful. Deliver me from self-reliance and stagnancy. Thank you for being faithful to keep your covenant despite my faults. Help me to spend time confessing your faithfulness so that I may trust in you wholeheartedly. Send your Spirit to help me take small steps toward you. Cultivate righteousness, justice, steadfast love, and compassion in me that I may model your faithfulness.

Suffer Faithfully

Blair Linne

Read

> But the Lord GOD helps me;
>> therefore I have not been disgraced;
>> therefore I have set my face like a flint,
>> and I know that I shall not be put to shame. (Isa. 50:7)

Reflect

One of my favorite places to go when I lived in Southern California was the Santa Monica Mountains. I set out hiking the dirt path that had long been traveled by those who walked or biked before me. Eventually I ended up on a large rock cliff that allowed me to look out over the Pacific Ocean. It was a stunning view. I had the Santa Monica Pier to my left, Malibu to my right, and a vast ocean that seemed to never end in front of me. I stood in awe as I beheld God's creation. The thought of making it to that rock cliff to behold the beauty motivated me despite the dangers that lurked in those mountains. I easily could've faced a mountain lion, a Pacific rattlesnake, or a twisted ankle. But time after time, I set those fears aside for a view of the beautiful landscape.

Jesus also encountered danger for the sake of a reward on a mountain: Golgotha, a skull-shaped hill in Jerusalem. In today's verse, we see that this mountain was where Jesus's face was set. Not because there was beauty immediately awaiting on that hilltop—there was a cross waiting. And unlike the mountain I climbed with a well-worn path of fellow travelers, Jesus was walking a path that no one else would or could.

How did he do it? He set his face like flint, like a hardened stone. In other words, Jesus had a firm resolution. He faithfully accepted the call he received from God. As we discussed yesterday, faithfulness grows in the face of resistance. Jesus knew he would face vexing trials. Not only was he misunderstood, mocked, denied, betrayed, and susceptible to physical and emotional harm; he would face God's wrath as he went to the cross as a sacrifice for sin! However, he was determined to live out the purpose that God set for him. Why? Because he trusted his father's character and word even above his circumstances.

Long before the world was created, God had a plan to exalt his Son. Part of that plan was redeeming mankind and all of creation through a loving covenant. What God promised was the truth that Christ trusted. Jesus knew his story wouldn't end on the chapter titled "Death." Therefore, Jesus endured the cross for the joy set before him. He saw life from an eternal perspective. He knew his resurrection and reign were still to come.

When we are suffering, Jesus shows us what it means to hold fast to God's covenant: We walk by faith and not by sight. We trust that God will use our small steps of obedience on the hard road of suffering to make us more like Christ and to bring us to glory.

Respond

Read James 1:12 and Revelation 2:10. How can you be faithful to God when he seems distant, or when you are weary? What is the reward for faithfully following our heavenly Father when faced with suffering or even death?

Request

Faithful Father, you are the God of glory. And yet you ordain suffering. Thank you for sending Jesus as the atoning Lamb to be the substitutionary sacrifice for my sins. Jesus suffered temporarily so I would not have to suffer eternally. God, help me when I suffer to remember Jesus. Let me be faithful in life and death.

Don't Wear the Faithfulness Mask

Blair Linne

Read

Woe to you, scribes and Pharisees, hypocrites! For you tithe mint and dill and cumin, and have neglected the weightier matters of the law: justice and mercy and faithfulness. These you ought to have done, without neglecting the others. (Matt. 23:23)

Reflect

When I was nine years old, my Saturdays were spent at the William Grant Still Arts Center learning theater acting along with other inner-city kids. We played improv games, rehearsed scenes, learned to project, and memorized monologues. For that hour or so on stage, we used all our training to pretend to be someone we were not.

In our text today, Jesus calls the scribes and Pharisees hypocrites. *Hypocrite* originates from a Greek word that means "actor" or "stage player." Jesus is calling these leaders out for wearing a mask over the heart. They were playing a role of faithfulness without possessing an inward heart of faith. These religious leaders were strict in outward practices that allowed them to be viewed positively. They honored God with their lips, but their hearts were far from him (Isa. 29:13).

When it's tempting to put on a faithfulness mask, pretending to be more than we are, we need to remember that God knows our hearts. Since faith is about placing an active trust in him, masquerading as outwardly faithful will never impact who we are inwardly. Pretending will never accomplish the goal of genuine faithfulness. Jesus wants actions that flow from hearts full of faith. If we lack inward faithfulness, we can ask him to transform us. God is a merciful God. When we humbly come to him acknowledging our lack of faith and asking him to work in us a faithfulness that we do not now possess, he gives grace.

Faithfulness is about worship. What or whom we deem worthy of worship challenges our *why*. Why are we obeying? Faithfulness is obedience that flows from a heart that has experienced God's presence. Thus when a faithful God commands us to love God with all our heart, soul, mind, and strength and our neighbor as ourselves, this must be prized as a matter worthy of our attention since it is the continuation of the faith we already possess. We cannot put these two commands on as if we are a stage actor in costume. We must appeal to God's supernatural power to obey his word genuinely. We prioritize worshiping God in private and worshiping with his people in the church. We protect the oppressed and show compassion to "the least of these" (Matt. 25:40). Our hearts break for the lost. And we recognize that every act of faithfulness is done only through God's power at work in us and for an audience of one.

Respond

Is there an area of your life where you are tempted to act outwardly more spiritual than you are internally? What would it look like for you to value inward obedience to God over outward signs that impress others?

Request

God of truth and compassion, I glorify you for your faithful commands. Lord, help me to be devoted to you wholeheartedly and to love my neighbor completely. May I prioritize having a heart that fully loves and obeys you in all things. Help me to obey your word even if others don't.

Faithfulness Isn't a Lonely Fruit

Blair Linne

Read

Yet I will leave seven thousand in Israel, all the knees that have
not bowed to Baal, and every mouth that has not kissed him.
(1 Kings 19:18)

Reflect

Elijah was a faithful prophet representing the true God amid a
people who worshiped false gods. The leaders of these false gods
had forsaken God's covenant. Because of this, they destroyed
God's altars and killed his prophets.

Elijah challenged King Ahab, Jezebel's husband, to gather the
false prophets to determine whose God was true. On his own,
Elijah contested the 450 prophets of Baal and Asherah. These
false prophets cried out to their god from morning until noon,
hoping for a fire to consume their bull offering. What did they
get in return? Silence. Finally, Elijah built his altar and poured

water over the offering (making it even more difficult to catch fire). He prayed to the true and living God. What happened? God sent fire to burn the bull offering, and the entire altar including the water was consumed. So Elijah proved to Ahab the true God from the false god.

Elijah was jealous for the Lord's name to be rightly honored, and the people's continued unfaithfulness—even after the stunning display of God's power—discouraged him. In his dismay, Elijah told the Lord that he was the only faithful prophet left (1 Kings 19:10).

To his great surprise, God told Elijah that he wasn't alone. God had reserved seven thousand in Israel who had not bowed to Baal. I'm sure that caused Elijah's mouth to gape. Seven thousand? From his vantage point, he was the only one being pursued and persecuted. But Elijah wasn't the only one who was faithful. There was a remnant God had preserved.

Like Elijah, we are not alone in our faithfulness. God is working in many places, preserving a diversely devoted people for himself who hold fast to his word. And, like Elijah, his people stand for what is true even when it's not popular.

One way we display that we are faithful to God is our faithfulness to the church. We do this by not neglecting to meet together (Heb. 10:25) and by looking out for the spiritual and physical good of the members of the church (Phil. 2:4). Faithfulness is our loyalty to God's gracious covenant, and God's covenant has been made for a body of believers, not merely one individual. God set it up that our growth and thriving in Christ is dependent upon us being a part of his body, the church.

As we surround ourselves with those who are faithful, it encourages our own faithfulness. When we are tempted to lose sight of

God's character or to believe that his promises are not intended for us, brothers and sisters in Christ remind us of what is true.

They also are a great help when we find ourselves feeling isolated like Elijah did. Christian community reminds us that we are not alone. We have a faithful God who loves us and has surrounded us with other faithful believers who will not bow down to idols but will faithfully serve the true and living God and encourage us to be faithful in the process.

Respond

Have you ever felt like you are the only one who is being faithful? In what ways has that been discouraging or disheartening to you? Take a few moments to consider those in your life who faithfully walk with God as an example for you to follow. How can you encourage them today? How can you be an example of faithfulness to others?

I can be faithful to the local church by _____

_____

I can be faithful to the global church by _____

_____

I can be faithful to my family by _____

_____

I can be faithful to my friends by _____

_____

I can be faithful to my enemies by _____

_____

Request

Gracious, covenant-keeping God, all blessing, honor, and faithfulness belong to you. Cleanse me from the pride of individualism and the temptation to think more highly of myself than I ought. Help me to be faithful toward the image bearers and believers you have placed in my life. Humble me by giving me mature saints who can correct me and sharpen me so that I may honor you in my faithfulness.

Blackberry and Plum Jam
Melissa Kruger

When we lived in Cambridge, England, my friend Stephanie knew of an open field that was full of blackberries. She also knew that the plum tree in my backyard was full of fruit. After picking bags and bags of fruit, she came over to my house and taught me to make jam. Both blackberries and plums have enough naturally occurring pectin so that this recipe works for either fruit or a combination of both. I've found that making jam is more of an art than a science and is most fun when a friend joins you for a chat while standing by the stove.

Ingredients

- 5 cups fruit (blackberries or plums)
- 2½ cups sugar (or more, depending upon how sweet you want it to be; increasing the sugar will also cause it to jam faster and result in a higher yield)
- 1 tablespoon lemon juice

Instructions

- Place a small plate in the freezer. Combine all ingredients in a medium saucepan and let sit for 10–15 minutes (or a couple of hours) without heat.

- Set stovetop heat to medium-low and simmer the jam for about 5–10 minutes until fruit mixture increasingly liquifies, stirring to keep the bubbles down. Skim off foam as needed. Use an immersion blender to blend mixture. Continue to heat on medium-low for 20–30 minutes, stirring constantly with a wooden spoon. You'll notice that the mixture will start to thicken and cling more to the spoon. After 25 minutes, put some jam on the plate from the freezer and wait 1 minute. If the mixture begins to solidify and doesn't run, the jam is ready. If it remains runny, continue to heat the jam for 5 more minutes and then repeat the test.

- Once jam is ready, pour into jars or containers and let them cool, making sure to leave room at the top if you plan to freeze. Let the mixture solidify overnight in the refrigerator. Whatever jam you don't plan to use in the next few weeks, put in the freezer for later.

- Note: I've made a lot of jams that were too runny (the result of not enough time on the stove) or too hard (too much time on the stove). These happy accidents can still be used. Runny jam makes a great topping for ice cream, oatmeal, or scones. Overly hard jam can be heated in the microwave for a minute to make it spreadable.

GENTLESS

We are apt to think that [Christ], being so holy, is therefore of a severe and sour disposition against sinners, and not able to bear them. "No," says he; "I am meek; gentleness is my name and temper."

THOMAS GOODWIN[11]

The Spirit Makes Us Gentle

Trillia Newbell

Read

Take my yoke upon you, and learn from me, for I am gentle and lowly in heart, and you will find rest for your souls. (Matt. 11:29)

Reflect

When I was thirteen years old, I rounded a corner on my bike, lost control, and slid across the concrete, leaving a layer of my skin on the ground. It was the worst wreck I've experienced (and that's saying a lot since I have been in a car accident). Thankfully, I wasn't too far from home. When I wobbled my way to my porch—crying from the pain and annoyance that my bike was now ruined—my mom came out and immediately scooped me up in her arms. Her concern was to care for me. She cleansed my wounds, helped me calm down, and never once mentioned my broken bike. In that moment, I needed my mother's gentleness.

Ultimately, cultivating the fruit of the Spirit means seeking to be transformed into the image of Christ. Today's text invites us to learn from our gentle Savior.

To be gentle is to be mild or humble. This might be surprising. We can understand Jesus as humble, but mild? Mild sounds weak or passive like a doormat. When I think of someone as mild, I think of shrinking back; I imagine a wimpy man or woman. But that's not a true characterization. Mildness is gentleness, and gentleness is godly. A gentle person extends forgiveness and mercy to others—even to those who are clearly in the wrong.

Gentleness can also be described by what it's not. It's not severe or harsh. A gentle person isn't easily provoked. A gentle person is not cruel. Gentleness reflects our Lord and Savior and is something we can emulate by the grace of God and the power of the Spirit.

As I look at descriptions of gentleness, I realize immediately where I fall short. I can be insensitive and demanding of those closest to me. I can be easily provoked and frustrated if I think someone is in the wrong. I can be insensitive, and my tongue can be unlovingly direct. Maybe you relate. Do you think about gentleness and feel conviction? The good news is, God always gives us the grace we need to change. As today's verse teaches us, Jesus's yoke is easy and his burden is light. We can run to him, confess our sin, and receive his help to become gentle.

Maybe reading this reflection has made you think about what you must do to change. But today, start with asking the Lord to do the work. Pray to be more like our gentle and mild Savior.

Respond

When you consider the definition of *gentleness*, where do you see a need to grow? Thinking about the life of Jesus, can you think of specific ways you can see his gentleness?

Request

Lord, thank you that you are a gentle Savior. Thank you that your yoke is easy and your burden is light. I confess that I am not always gentle. I can be harsh with my words and unkind with my private thoughts. Thank you that you tell me that if I confess my sin, you are faithful and just to forgive me and purify me. Jesus, thank you!

Suffering People Need
a Gentle Savior

Trillia Newbell

Read

> But the woman, knowing what had happened to her, came in fear
> and trembling and fell down before him and told him the whole
> truth. And he said to her, "Daughter, your faith has made you
> well; go in peace, and be healed of your disease." (Mark 5:33–34)

Reflect

During the height of the Covid pandemic, my mom spent three
weeks in the hospital. No one was allowed to visit her. All we could
do was call and pray. She appreciated our prayers and believed
that God heard every one of them, but she missed our presence.
When she healed, we were so grateful to have her home, but her
fight wasn't over, and neither was her isolation.

We all know people who are suffering in various ways. Some
are suffering from chronic illness. Others, like my mom, are

suffering from sickness that comes on quickly and lingers for a long time. And even more are experiencing invisible suffering that happens only in the mind. Jesus gently cared for people under every category of human suffering we can imagine. In today's verses, we see his gentleness when he interacted with the woman with a discharge of blood.

Jesus had just stepped out of a boat when a great crowd began to gather and then follow him (Mark 5:21–24). A woman who had been bleeding for twelve years was among the people eager to be near Jesus. She was suffering not only physically but financially too. She had been to many physicians, and no one had helped her. She was out of money, and I imagine she was running out of hope for healing as well (v. 26). The significance of her bleeding meant that she was essentially untouchable. She would have been considered ceremonially unclean (Lev. 15:25–28). Everyone who touched her also became unclean (Lev. 15:19). Can you imagine her sense of isolation? And her deep desire to find healing?

In her desperation, she reached out to touch Jesus's garment. She believed he could heal her.

While others might have shied away from the woman—fearing that her uncleanness would make them unclean—Jesus affection-ally called her "daughter." He reached out in gentleness and wel-comed her into his family—the family of God! He acknowledged her faith and declared her well. We can assume that the famil-ial language coupled with the declaration of "well" rather than "healed" means she was both physically and spiritually made well.

Although we can't physically heal others, our response to their suffering does matter. We can communicate with gentleness and compassion, or we can respond in a way that alienates and belittles.

In today's passage, the Lord was not annoyed, frustrated, or angry. He didn't rebuke the woman. He was gentle and loving, tender and kind. Because of his great mercy and grace toward us, we can extend gentleness to others.

Respond

In what ways does suffering isolate us from others? What would it look like to respond in gentleness and compassion to those who are suffering? How can you bring your struggles and trials today to Jesus (i.e., "touch his garment in faith")? How can you entrust those hardships to him in new ways?

Request

Lord, help me to be slow to speak, gentle, and patient. Help me to gain empathy. Thank you, Jesus, that you were tempted in every way and are sympathetic to those enduring trials of various kinds. Jesus, help me to bring my every burden to you.

Gentleness Is Your Calling

Trillia Newbell

Read

> I therefore, a prisoner for the Lord, urge you to walk in a manner worthy of the calling to which you have been called, with all humility and gentleness, with patience, bearing with one another in love, eager to maintain the unity of the Spirit in the bond of peace. (Eph. 4:1–3)

Reflect

When I think about the calling the Lord has given me as a follower of Jesus, I often think of big things. I'm called to make disciples, to share the gospel and teach others to obey. I'm called to be a committed wife and mom. I'm called to be a faithful church member. I'm called to do my work to the glory of the Lord. All of these things are important. However, I must admit that until recently, I'd never thought about how gentleness is a part of my call.

If you've placed your trust in the finished work of Jesus, you and I have the same call. We're called to obey God with our heart, mind, soul, and strength, and to love our neighbors as ourselves. Our calling is to walk in a manner worthy of what we've received. We've received Christ's righteousness and ought to walk worthy of that gift.

Gentleness is part of our calling because gentleness displays the gospel to our neighbors. Our gentleness toward one another is important because it points to the one who lived and died for us. By his grace we can be gentle toward each other. As we remind ourselves of the gift we've received, we can pray that the overflow of our transformed hearts would reflect the gentleness of our Savior.

There are endless ways we can apply the gentleness we see in Christ to our own lives and the way that we interact with others. But perhaps the most striking and clear connection to the gospel is how we correct and restore those who confess sin. Paul tells us in Galatians 6:1, "Brothers, if anyone is caught in any transgression, you who are spiritual should restore him in a spirit of gentleness. Keep watch on yourself, lest you too be tempted." There is a call here to love your neighbor as yourself and treat the person caught in sin as you'd want to be treated. To restore isn't to ignore someone's sin (just as the gospel doesn't ignore our sin). Instead, we are to correct or admonish, which if done in gentleness (humility) can lead to restoration.

Aren't we glad God didn't treat us as our sins deserved? We should do likewise. God doesn't ignore our sin. Neither should we ignore our neighbor's sin. But if we understand the depths of sin that we have been forgiven, we will restore our neighbor with gentleness and humility. We will display the same grace we've received from our Lord.

Jesus told his disciples that people would know we are his disciples by our love for one another (John 13:35). One outworking of our love for one another is our gentleness toward one another. It matters because it is about our Lord, not about us. So today we ask the Lord to help us walk in a manner worthy of the grace we've received and display the gentleness of our Lord to all.

Respond

Take a moment to consider the various callings you've been given: relationally, vocationally, spiritually. In what ways could you be gentle in those callings? How is gentleness different from the way the world usually works? Why is being gentle such a witness to the watching world?

Request

Lord, I know that I am not always gentle with those around me. I know that it can be easy to see the sin in others and hold it against them. Help me to remember your grace. Help me to grow in humility and love. Thank you for your great mercy that has made a way for me and those around me to know you.

Gentleness Helps Others Honor God

Trillia Newbell

Read

A soft answer turns away wrath,
    but a harsh word stirs up anger. (Prov. 15:1)

Reflect

I'm not afraid of conflict. I often run straight toward it. Although I don't know the psychology behind my response, I do know that when I've allowed my flesh to take over, my fighting instinct hasn't always been beneficial. Sadly, my words are often sharp, critical, harsh, and quick. When I lack self-control with my tongue, I'm the opposite of gentle. And if I'm not wise with my words and gentle in my speech, my not-so-soft answer will receive the response we see here in our text: anger.

Today's verse—one I often meditate on—helps us learn how to speak and examine our words. Interestingly, it shows that our words not only affect others, but how we speak also benefits us! Although the ESV uses the word *soft*, many translations use the word *gentle*. This proverb isn't suggesting that we speak quietly (although that's better than screaming); this verse exposes the power of our tongues to evoke a sinful response in others. Sin is never done in isolation. In other words, when we sin against someone, it often tempts the other person to sin. Our sin always affects others in one way or another.

I once heard a story about a woman who had a habit of assuming her husband's motives and believing the worst. One night she yelled at him, "Why do you always do this? You never put away socks!" It seems like a minor issue, but to her, it meant he was lazy and uncaring. Her husband took the socks, threw them in the drawer, and then yelled back, "Those aren't even mine!" That's right, they were her socks! He struggled to speak to her for most of the night.

He felt angry, accused, and belittled. You can imagine how *she* felt. But what might have happened if she slowed down, took a deep breath, and believed the best about her husband? Even if she didn't look closely at the socks, it would have changed the whole night if she had spoken kindly even in her error. But she spoke in anger and accusation. She sinned. Then he sinned. All of it was avoidable. Guarding our tongues helps others honor our Lord.

The reality of living in a fallen world is that there will be times when you and I give a gentle answer but still receive an angry response. We can't control the actions of others. But because of Jesus, we have a way of escape (1 Cor. 10:13). You and I don't have to sin. We can say no. We can control our own actions. We have the power of the Spirit to resist the urge to do what our flesh (sin nature) wants us to do. And when we speak gently to others, we bless them, and we also and ultimately honor our Lord.

Respond

Read Proverbs 10:19; 12:18; and 17:27. What warnings do these proverbs offer about how we use our words? Have you ever lost control of your tongue and said something you wish you hadn't? How did the other person respond? Now think of a time when you were gentle. How did that go?

Request

Dear Lord, help me guard my tongue. When I speak unkindly, help me to remember that my sin affects those around me. Grow me in the fear of the Lord that I might worship you and speak in a manner that honors you. Lord, you are faithful; you will surely do it.

Winter Fruit Salad with Lemon-Poppyseed Dressing
Megan Hill

I received this recipe from my pastor's wife when I was engaged to be married. Her example of hospitality and this trusty recipe gave me confidence to welcome people into my home.

Ingredients

Salad:
- 1 head romaine lettuce, shredded
- 4 ounces (1 cup) shredded Monterey Jack cheese
- 1 cup cashews
- ½ cup dried cranberries
- 1 apple, diced
- 1 pear, diced

Dressing:
- ⅓ cup sugar
- ⅓ cup lemon juice
- 2 teaspoons chopped onion
- 1 teaspoon Dijon mustard
- ½ teaspoon salt
- 1 tablespoon poppy seeds
- ⅔ cup vegetable oil

Instructions

- Toss all salad ingredients in a large bowl.

- Combine all dressing ingredients except oil in blender or food processor. Add oil slowly while machine is running.

- Pour over salad and toss to combine.

SELF-CONTROL

Let not that man think he makes any progress
in holiness who walks not over the bellies of
his lusts. He who doth not kill sin in this way
takes no steps toward his journey's end.

JOHN OWEN[12]

Learn to Say No

Sharonda Cooper

Read

Every athlete exercises self-control in all things. They do it to receive a perishable wreath, but we an imperishable. (1 Cor. 9:25)

Reflect

What is self-control? As the final attribute in Paul's list of the Spirit's fruit, it holds a place of significance. By definition, it refers to the ability to control one's desires. It's the thing that helps you keep those New Year's resolutions. It's the thing that gets you out of bed when you want to hit snooze a third time. It's what you feel is missing in the comments section of many internet posts these days. In a nutshell, it's the ability to say no when your flesh is saying yes.

The Bible emphasizes a few specific applications of self-control. The first is sexual purity. Paul commands Christians to abstain from sexual immorality by learning how to "control [their] own body in holiness and honor, not in the passion of lust like the Gentiles who do not know God" (1 Thess. 4:4). For the unmarried woman, this means abstinence. For the married woman, this means upholding the sanctity of the marriage bed. A lack of self-control leaves single women prone to promiscuity and married women prone to infidelity.

A second facet of self-control relates to stewardship of our bodies. In today's verse, Paul uses the example of a runner who must exercise self-control in all things. If the athlete fails to do so and gives in to every tempting milkshake or slice of pizza, he can kiss the gold medal goodbye. The language used in 1 Corinthians 9:27 is compelling: "But I discipline my body and keep it under control." The runner's desire to win compels him not only to train hard, but also to refuse unwholesome food, alcohol, or other indulgences. First Corinthians 6:19 reminds us that our bodies are the temple of the Holy Spirit. While there are certainly times for joyful feasting, habitual excess with food and drink may signify gluttony (Prov. 23:20). A lifestyle focused on ease and comfort may lead to sloth. Self-control is the tool we use to keep the dangers of fleshly indulgence at bay.

A third facet of self-control in Scripture is Christlike speech. The wise one knows, "Whoever keeps his mouth and his tongue keeps himself out of trouble" (Prov. 21:23). If only this were the banner across every social-media feed. Christians need not be taught that the tongue is a fire (James 3:6). It's obvious. We tell our teen son, "Just because it's true doesn't mean you need to say it." Yet I find it so hard to hold back my running commentary when we watch the evening news. I am often critical and far too quick to judge. Self-control helps us avoid saying things we might later regret.

Ultimately, self-control is saying no to one thing and yes to something better. Obedience to Christ is better than sexual sin, the tastiest meal, or a snarky comment. When we exhibit self-control, we testify to a self-indulgent world that Jesus is better.

Respond

Read Genesis 3:1–7. What were the steps leading up to Eve's sinful act? What three things did she see about the tree that caused her to take of its fruit? What does this account teach you about self-control? How can you learn from Eve's mistake?

As you think about self-control, in what ways does it impact all the other fruit we've studied so far? Is there an area you are struggling right now with self-control? When is self-control particularly difficult for you?

Request

Heavenly Father, I confess that I often give in to sinful desires. I choose what I want over what is best, and I sometimes value comfort a little too much. Just this week I have made some poor choices. Please forgive me. Teach me to be the kind of woman who will not let sinful desires hijack my obedience. Help me learn to say no to harmful or simply unhelpful things. Holy Spirit, please grow the fruit of self-control in my heart so that my life will bring honor to the name of Christ.

Only Eat the Best Bread

Sharonda Cooper

Read

Jesus said to them, "My food is to do the will of him who sent me and to accomplish his work." (John 4:34)

Reflect

Have you ever noticed that life is harder when you're hungry? Most days I wake up and have nothing but water and black coffee until noon. This means morning is not the best time for me to deal with angry drivers, check my social-media account, or take notice of the laundry sprawled on my son's bedroom floor. When I'm hungry, I'm just much more likely to say and do the wrong thing.

Early in Jesus's ministry he was tempted by the devil in the wilderness. After forty days of fasting Jesus was hungry. We can only imagine! At this opportune time the tempter said, "If you are the Son of God, command these stones to become loaves of bread"

(Matt. 4:3). Satan figured Jesus was hungry enough to abandon the mission God entrusted to him. Thankfully, Satan was wrong.

Jesus's response indicates that he desired to glorify God more than he wanted a meal. He said, "It is written, 'Man shall not live by bread alone, but by every word that comes from the mouth of God'" (Matt. 4:4). It would have been easy for him to say the word and turn the stone into bread. But by denying himself, he taught us something about self-control: sometimes we must forgo the thing that *feels* good so we can have the thing that *is* good.

It's difficult to say no to things that bring immediate pleasure. Sexual sin may bring temporary satisfaction. An extra glass of wine might seem like the perfect reward after a long day with the kids. Taking a verbal swipe at a coworker might make you feel vindicated in a meeting. All these things serve the flesh but fail to tell the truth about the thing of greatest worth. We can learn from Christ's response in today's verse. His mission was to do his Father's will, so he joyfully rejected anything that would get in the way. Turning the stone into bread was not the Father's will, so Christ rejected Satan's offer.

On the other hand, eating bread when you're hungry isn't always sinful. Jesus ate plenty of bread on other occasions. Furthermore, food miracles were not the issue either—he later turned water into wine and multiplied fishes and loaves. However, in this moment, God had called Jesus to fast. Through his hunger, Jesus was able to identify with our suffering. And he obeyed in spite of his hunger.

How was Jesus able to exhibit such self-control? The secret lies in understanding his highest goal. He wanted to eat, but he wanted something else even more. He was hungry for God's glory.

His food was to do the will of God (John 4:34). When bringing glory to Christ is our greatest desire, we can say no to anything that jeopardizes that goal. The athlete turns down the pizza the night before a race because he wants to win.

To cultivate self-control, we look to Jesus as our example. He was tempted but did not sin because he cherished God's glory more than anything else. Perhaps this is why he told us to love God with all our heart, soul, strength, and mind (Luke 10:27). If we are honest, we must admit that we often fail to love God supremely. Thankfully, God promises by his Holy Spirit to give us more love, new desires, and the self-control to bring him glory in all we say and do. That's really good news.

Respond

Read Isaiah 53:7–9, which mentions another time Jesus exhibited self-control. What event is the prophet referring to in this passage (see Matt. 26:57–68)? Now continue reading, Isaiah 53:10–12, to find out *why* Jesus endured such suffering. Knowing that Jesus could have responded differently, how does his humble silence encourage you?

Request

Gracious Lord, I struggle to exhibit self-control when it comes to _____. I know that I should _____, but I often _____. Second Timothy 1:7 says you have given me the spirit of self-control. Please help me to live in light of that truth. Spirit, as I look to Christ, please help me to reject anything that will stand in the way of my making much of his name. Make me a woman who is self-controlled for your glory and my good.

Self-Control Keeps You Safe

Sharonda Cooper

Read

A man without self-control
    is like a city broken into and left without walls. (Prov. 25:28)

Reflect

When I was a little girl, our apartment was robbed. Items were moved, drawers were left opened, and many things were just gone. Our front door, with all its locks and bolts, had not protected us. I remember how I felt when we arrived home that day. I felt violated. I felt angry. But most of all, I felt unsafe. The things designed to protect us had failed.

The writers of the proverbs often use similes to help us understand truths about life. Our verse today is a proverb that compares a man to a city and self-control to the city's walls. City walls are designed to protect. A city without walls is vulnerable and unsafe—just like my family was the day we were robbed.

It's easy to understand this concept in the context of sexual temptation. A lack of self-control led King David to adultery and murder (2 Sam. 11). Solomon's polygamy led to idolatry (1 Kings 11:1–3). And Samson's obsession with Philistine women cost him his eyes and eventually his life (Judg. 16). But there are other ways that a lack of self-control can leave us vulnerable. Think of the young mom who spends so much time scrolling through internet pictures that she misses precious opportunities with her children, or the grandmother whose sweet tooth leads to deteriorating health, or the church member whose tendency to gossip destroys her friendships. Without self-control, we are like a city without walls—an easy target for attack.

Have you heard about the research study of children playing soccer? In this study, the children who were given no rules had no fun. Without structure, nothing is fair and no one knows what to do. On the other hand, the children with rules and a referee had a blast. Boundaries provide freedom to play the game.

Self-control is a gift that allows us to be free to live as God intends. We are no longer forced to obey our passions. As Paul reminds us in Romans 6:6–7, "We know that our old self was crucified with him in order that the body of sin might be brought to nothing, so that we would no longer be enslaved to sin. For one who has died has been set free from sin." When sin calls us back to bondage, self-control guards our freedom.

Once my parents realized that someone had been in our apartment, they immediately called the police. The next day the locks were changed on our front door, but I never felt safe there again. It has been over thirty-five years since that horrible day, and I now live in a safe, quiet neighborhood, but I still feel insecure without all our doors locked and our house alarm activated. Early in our marriage I told my husband that he could help me feel safe by being the last one to lock up at bedtime. When he comes to bed, I'm free to rest. The doors are locked, the alarm is on, and it won't be easy for an intruder to get inside.

According to Scripture, cultivating self-control is like putting up a protective wall. When presented with sin, we have the self-control to resist it. We have the Spirit! And where the Spirit of the Lord is, there is freedom (2 Cor. 3:17).

Respond

Second Peter 2:19 teaches, "Whatever overcomes a person, to that he is enslaved." Are there unhelpful behaviors you struggle to eliminate from your life? Do you spend too much time, money, or effort on things that prevent you from obeying God? Write down one or two things you feel have too much of a hold on you. Imagine how your life would change if you could control your desires in those areas.

Request

Dear Lord, I confess that I have trouble saying no to _____. Please forgive me for allowing my desires to control me. I want to grow in holiness, and this is getting in the way. I do not want to be a slave to anything but you. Spirit, help me cultivate self-control so that I can be free to live a life of obedience and holiness for the glory of Christ.

Self-Control Bears Fruit

Sharonda Cooper

Read

His divine power has granted to us all things that pertain to life and godliness. . . . For this very reason, make every effort to supplement your faith with virtue, and virtue with knowledge, and knowledge with self-control, and self-control with steadfastness, and steadfastness with godliness, and godliness with brotherly affection, and brotherly affection with love. For if these qualities are yours and are increasing, they keep you from being ineffective or unfruitful in the knowledge of our Lord Jesus Christ. (2 Pet. 1:3, 5–8)

Reflect

We have some family friends—a sweet couple—who had been out of church for years. As they sat on our sofa one afternoon, my husband and I asked them about their reasons for neglecting to gather with the body of Christ. They gave excuse after excuse until I asked questions that left them speechless. "How are you being obedient to the 'one another' passages of Scripture? How are you pouring into the lives of other believers?" I asked. After a long pause the husband said, "I guess we're not."

Those friends of ours are faithfully serving in a local church today, but at the time, they simply had not considered the effect their personal decisions could have on others. Sometimes we think that way about self-control. We think we can sin without hurting anyone else, but a lack of self-control can wreak havoc in the lives of others. Gossip can kill a friendship (Prov. 16:28), yet we still sometimes let a friend's private information slip out in the form of a prayer request. Obsession with your phone can make the person across the table feel like they're your last priority. Harsh words stir up anger among us (Prov. 15:1), but it's so easy to be short with those we love. Self-control applies to all forms of fleshly desires and passions—including the propensity to say or do the wrong thing at the wrong time in the wrong way.

Not only can a lack of self-control affect our relationships with other believers; it can also affect our witness. My daughter is a college freshman, and she has been shocked by the rampant promiscuity on her campus. The university's administrators assume that college students have no self-control whatsoever. Sex is treated like a bodily function—like an itch that must be scratched. But we are made in God's image and are not like the animals. The world needs to see people who are not controlled by fleshly lusts and desires. So when a Christian college student holds her tongue as a professor ridicules her worldview, or when she refuses to take a shot of liquor just because everyone else is doing it, or when she commits to a lifestyle of sexual abstinence, she's telling unbelievers something about God and something about humanity. The self-controlled person stands out in a society that's out of control.

Have you ever wondered why self-control is the last listed fruit of the Spirit? Perhaps self-control helps us cultivate all the other fruit.

When I am self-controlled, I can:

- be free to *love* others more than myself;
- find *joy* in the Lord instead of in online gossip;
- stop overindulging in news that steals my *peace* and makes me fearful of tomorrow;
- choose not to raise my voice in anger but have *patience* with my teammate;
- show *kindness* even to the angry neighbor across the street;
- demonstrate *goodness* by taking the time to disciple a young mom in the church;
- maintain *faithfulness* to my husband even when my male coworker's advances go too far;
- speak with *gentleness* when I must rebuke someone for sin.

Self-control, in a sense, provides the atmosphere for all the other areas of the fruit to grow. Just as a tree will bear fruit when it is protected from harm, our lives will bear fruit when we have the self-control to reject the things that can destroy us. Today's passage encourages us to pursue self-control so we will live effective lives that are a blessing to others. Friends, God has given us everything we need (2 Pet. 1:3). As we turn away from our sin and look to

Christ, the Holy Spirit will produce in us the self-controlled life that glorifies the holy name of our great God.

Respond

Read James 1:19 and list the three commands given. How do these behaviors benefit relationships between people? How would cultivating self-control help you live out this text in your family? Your church? With unbelievers in your life?

Request

Father, thank you for helping me understand the importance of self-control. I confess that my poor choices sometimes affect my relationships with others and make it hard for unbelievers to notice anything different about me. Help me, Holy Spirit, to bear fruit in this area. Teach me to reject any behaviors that fail to bring honor to your name.

Perfect Cranberry Sauce

Megan Hill

This makes an appearance at our table every Thanksgiving. Make an extra batch so you have plenty for next-day leftovers!

Makes 2 cups

Ingredients

- 1 bag (12 ounces) fresh or frozen cranberries, rinsed
- 1 cup sugar
- 1 orange, zested and juiced
- ¾ teaspoon ground ginger or 1½ teaspoons freshly grated ginger

Instructions

- Combine cranberries, sugar, orange juice (save zest), and ginger in a dutch oven. Bring to boil over medium-high heat. Reduce heat to simmer. Once berries begin to pop (about 2 minutes), cover, turn off heat, and let stand for 10 minutes.

- Stir zest into sauce. Cool to room temperature and then refrigerate until cold.

Flourish with Fruit for Tomorrow

Melissa Kruger

Read

> The righteous flourish like the palm tree
>   and grow like a cedar in Lebanon.
> They are planted in the house of the LORD;
>   they flourish in the courts of our God.
> They still bear fruit in old age;
>   they are ever full of sap and green,
> to declare that the LORD is upright;
>   he is my rock, and there is no unrighteousness in him.
>   (Ps. 92:12–15)

Reflect

Last week I visited my daughter at her university, my alma mater. The campus looked just as I remembered it. We ate at my favorite frozen yogurt shop (now hers as well). I showed her the buildings where I had most of my classes. I pointed out the spot where her dad asked me out for the first time—thirty years ago.

Somehow, it feels like yesterday.

And yet when I catch a glimpse of myself in the mirror, I see an older woman staring back at me. I may feel just a few years older than my eighteen-year-old self, but in reality I'm closer to retirement age than college age. Sometimes, it's difficult to believe how quickly the years have gone by.

As I continue to gain more gray hairs and an increasing number of wrinkles, today's verses provide fresh encouragement. Outwardly my body may wear away, but inwardly I'm being renewed day by day. I don't have to fear becoming dry and brittle. God promises that the righteous will flourish—those planted in the house of the Lord will still bear fruit in old age.

How can I be confident in my righteousness? I'm confident because it's not mine. It's a gift. We can claim perfect righteousness, not because of our works, but because of Jesus. He who knew no sin became sin, that we might become the righteousness of God (2 Cor. 5:21). His body was broken, his blood was shed. He tasted death so that we might live.

Born by the Spirit, we belong in the house of the Lord. United with Christ, we are connected to his people, the church. We are not alone. We are daughters, sisters, mothers, grandmothers, and great-grandmothers in the family of God. No matter our age or marital status, we have opportunity to tell the next generation about the deeds of the Lord. We get to declare his goodness, to tell how he was the rock on which we stood firm when the rains came and the storm winds blew. Planted in his house, we flourish.

Thankfully, bearing fruit in old age doesn't involve expensive creams or procedures. Whatever our age, we're told that "those who look to him are radiant" (Ps. 34:5). As the years continue to pass, I hope to become a woman whose face crinkles with a joyful glow—one that comes from another year of knowing Christ and being increasingly conformed to his likeness. In a world that tells us our best days are behind us, the hope of knowing Christ reminds us that the best is yet to come. We have bright hope for tomorrow.

Respond

In what ways does this passage encourage you as you consider aging? In what ways can older believers bear fruit in younger believers' lives? What can you do today to connect with God's people in the church?

Request

Oh, Lord, I want to be a woman who bears an increasing harvest of fruit with each passing year. Plant me in your house and let me flourish in your courts. Thank you for making me righteous in Christ and giving me a home with your people. Bless me, that I might be a blessing to others all the days of my life.

Notes

1. Charles H. Spurgeon, "Herein Is Love," *Bible Commentaries: 1 John 4*, Spurgeon's Verse Expositions of the Bible, StudyLight.org, January 19, 1896, https://www.studylight.org/.

2. Paul E. Miller, *A Loving Life: In a World of Broken Relationships* (Wheaton, IL: Crossway, 2014), 43.

3. Frances Ridley Havergal, "The Abiding Joy," in *Seasons of the Heart: A Year of Devotions from One Generation of Women to Another*, ed. Donna Kelderman (Grand Rapids, MI: Reformation Heritage, 2013), January 11 entry.

4. Alexander MacLaren, *Expositions of Holy Scripture: Second Corinthians, Galatians, Philippians, Colossians, Thessalonians, and First Timothy* (Grand Rapids, MI: Eerdmans, 1932), 164.

5. Jay Sklar, *Numbers* (Grand Rapids, MI: Zondervan, 2023).

6. John Calvin, *Calvin's Commentaries*, vol. 19, *Acts 14–28; Romans 1–16* (1974; repr., Grand Rapids, MI: Baker, 1993), 310.

7. Charles H. Spurgeon, "Christ's People—Imitators of Him," in *New Park Street Pulpit Volume 1*, The Spurgeon Center for Biblical Preaching at Midwestern Seminary, accessed June 28, 2023, https://www.spurgeon.org/.

8. Richard Sibbes, "The Privileges of the Faithful," in *The Complete Works of Richard Sibbes* (Edinburgh: James Nichol, 1863), 5:282.

9. Thomas Lye, "Puritan Sermons," in *Voices from the Past*, ed. Richard Rushing (Edinburgh: Banner of Truth, 2009), 185; emphasis added.

10. Cited in Tim Hansel, *Holy Sweat: The Remarkable Things Ordinary People Can Do When They Let God Use Them* (Waco, TX: Word, 1987), 130.

11. Thomas Goodwin, *The Heart of Christ* (Carlisle, PA: Banner of Truth, 2011), 63.

12. John Owen, *The Mortification of Sin*, trans. Aaron M. Renn (New York: TradLife Press, 2019), 26.

Scripture Index

TGC THE GOSPEL COALITION

The Gospel Coalition (TGC) supports the church in making disciples of all nations, by providing gospel-centered resources that are trusted and timely, winsome and wise.

Guided by a Council of more than 40 pastors in the Reformed tradition, TGC seeks to advance gospel-centered ministry for the next generation by producing content (including articles, podcasts, videos, courses, and books) and convening leaders (including conferences, virtual events, training, and regional chapters).

In all of this we want to help Christians around the world better grasp the gospel of Jesus Christ and apply it to all of life in the 21st century. We want to offer biblical truth in an era of great confusion. We want to offer gospel-centered hope for the searching.

Through its women's initiatives, The Gospel Coalition aims to support the growth of women in faithfully studying and sharing the Scriptures; in actively loving and serving the church; and in spreading the gospel of Jesus Christ in all their callings.

Join us by visiting TGC.org so you can be equipped to love God with all your heart, soul, mind, and strength, and to love your neighbor as yourself.

TGC.org